MONITORING FLUID AND ELECTROLYTES PRECISELY

MONITORING FLUID AND ELECTROLYTES PRECISELY

Nursing80 Books
Intermed Communications, Inc.
Horsham, Pennsylvania

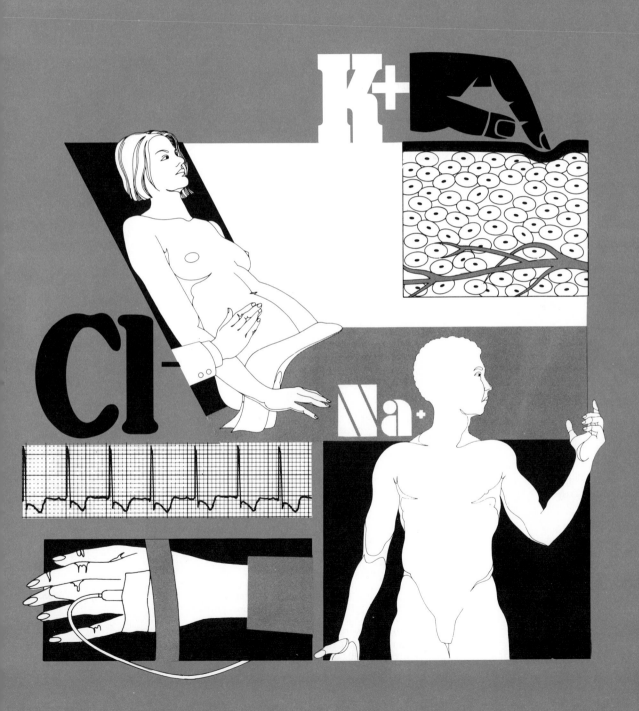

NURSING80® BOOKS

PUBLISHER: Eugene W. Jackson
Editorial Director: Daniel L. Cheney
Clinical Director: Margaret Van Meter, RN
Graphics Director: John Isely
General Manager: T. A. Temple

NURSING79 SKILLBOOK SERIES
Editorial staff for this volume:
Book Editor: Helen Hamilton
Clinical Editor: Minnie Rose, RN, BSN, MEd
Marginalia Editor: Avery Rome
Associate Clinical Editor: Catherine Manzi, RN
Nursing Consultant: Barbara McVan, RN
Copy Editors: Patricia Hamilton, Kathy Lorenc
Researcher and Indexer: Vonda Heller
Production Manager: Bernard Haas
Production Assistants: David C. Kosten, Margie Tyson
Designers: Maggie Arnott, Robert Jackson
Artists: Kim Milnazic, Robert Renn, and Sandra Simms

Clinical consultants
Nancy Blackburn, RN, BS, *Special Program Coordinator, Wilmington Medical Center, Wilmington, Del.*
Carol Kushner, RN, BSN, MSN, *Nursing Supervisor, Medical College of Pennsylvania, Philadelphia, Pa.*
Despina Seremelis, RN, BSN, *Staff Nurse, Temple University Hospital, Philadelphia, Pa.*
Mark Victor, MD, *Resident, Internal Medicine, Hahnemann Medical College and Hospital, Philadelphia, Pa.*

Fifth Printing.
Copyright © 1972, 1973, 1974, 1975, 1977, 1978, 1979
by Intermed Communications, Inc.
132 Welsh Road, Horsham, Pa. 19044

Library of Congress Cataloging in Publication Data
Main entry under title:

MONITORING FLUID AND ELECTROLYTES PRECISELY
"Nursing Skillbook series"
Bibliography: p. 208
Includes index.
1. Body fluid disorders. 2. Water-electrolyte imbalances.
3. Monitoring (hospital care). 4. Nursing.
[DNLM: 1. Water-electrolyte balance — Nursing texts.
2. Water-electrolyte imbalance — Nursing texts.
3. Monitoring, Physiologic — Nursing texts.   QU105 M744]
RC630.M65   616'.047   77-20636
ISBN 0-916730-09-3

CONTENTS

Guide to drug charts

The symbol ◇ after a trade name indicates that the drug is also available in Canada.

The symbol ◇◇ means that the drug is available in Canada only.

Unmarked trade names mean that the drug is available only in the United States.

These symbols will be used in all the drug charts throughout the book.

AUTHORS

Barbara A. Bonaventura is a staff development instructor for medical and critical care nursing at the Hospital of the Medical College of Pennsylvania, Philadelphia. She received her BSN from Temple University, Philadelphia.

Lavenia G. Coleman is director of intravenous therapy at Temple University Health Sciences Center, Philadelphia. She is a graduate of Kings County Hospital Center School of Nursing, Brooklyn, New York.

Rita Colley is a nurse clinician in hyperalimentation at Massachusetts General Hospital, Boston. She is a graduate of Massachusetts General Hospital School of Nursing and received a BA from the University of Massachusetts, Boston.

Diane K. Dressler, a staff nurse at St. Luke's Hospital, Milwaukee, received a BSN from the University of Wisconsin, Madison, and is presently a graduate student in nursing at Marquette University, Milwaukee, Wisconsin.

Nancy Elbaum is a staff nurse at St. John's Hospital, Santa Monica, California. She received her BSN from UCLA School of Nursing, Los Angeles.

Alice Gillis is presently doing independent study while working on a MSN from Marquette University, Milwaukee, Wisconsin. She received her BSN at Alderson-Broaddus College, Philippi, West Virginia.

Carol Ann Gramse is a full-time doctoral student at New York University, New York, where she also earned her MA. She is a BSN graduate of Hunter College-Bellevue School of Nursing, New York.

Ann P. Gregory is assistant professor of maternal-child nursing, College of Nursing, University of Delaware, Newark, Delaware. She received her BS from Wagner College, Staten Island, New York, and her MSN from the University of Pennsylvania, Philadelphia.

Stanley E. Grissinger is director of pharmacy service, Suburban General Hospital, Norristown, Pennsylvania. He received his BSc from Temple University, Philadelphia.

Claudella Archambeault Jones is educational director for the National Institute for Burn Medicine, Ann Arbor, Michigan. She is a graduate of the Mercy School of Nursing, Toledo, Ohio.

Louise M. Juliani is an instructor at the University of Texas School of Nursing. She received her BSN from the University of Wisconsin, Madison, and her MSN from Boston University, Boston.

Joyce L. Kee, assistant professor at the University of Delaware College of Nursing, Newark, received both her BSN and MSN at the University of Maryland, Baltimore. Ms. Kee is an advisor for *Nursing78*.

Jane Lancour is director of clinical nursing at St. Luke's Hospital and assistant clinical professor at Marquette University College of Nursing, Milwaukee. She is a graduate of St. John's Hospital School of Nursing, Springfield, Illinois, received her BSN and MSN from Marquette University, Milwaukee.

Carla Ann Lee, assistant professor and project director of the Nurse Clinical Program, Wichita State University, in Kansas is a graduate of St. Joseph School of Nursing, Salina, Kansas. She received her BSN at the University of Kansas, Lawrence, Kansas, and her MA at Wichita State University, Wichita.

Catherine Ciaverelli Manzi, an assistant editor for *Nursing78*, is a graduate of Hahnemann Hospital School of Nursing, Philadelphia.

Gretchen Reed is an instructor of anatomy and physiology at the University of Tennessee Center for the Health Sciences, Knoxville, and a charge nurse for Methodist Hospital Central, Cardiology Stepdown Unit, Memphis. Ms. Reed is presently a PhD candidate at the University of Tennessee, Knoxville.

Kathryn E. Richards is assistant professor of surgery and clinical instructor to the department of surgery, University of Michigan, Ann Arbor. She received her MD from the University of Michigan Medical School, Ann Arbor, Michigan.

Minnie Rose is a clinical editor for *Nursing78* Book Division. She received her BSN from Indiana University, Bloomington, Indiana, and her MEd from Temple University, Philadelphia.

June L. Stark is head nurse of the transplant unit, Boston Veterans' Hospital, Boston. She is a graduate of Jackson Memorial Hospital School of Nursing, Miami, Florida.

Hannelore Sweetwood, director of inservice education at Jersey Shore Medical Center, Neptune, New Jersey, is a graduate of Jersey City Medical Center School of Nursing, Jersey City. She received her BS and is a candidate for an MS in education at Monmouth College, West Long Branch, New Jersey.

Russell W. Thomas is a clinical pharmacist at Temple University Hospital, Philadelphia. He received his BSc in pharmacy at the Philadelphia College of Pharmacy and Science.

Marilyn Twombly, a certified enterostomal therapist, is a clinical nurse specialist at the Medical College of Wisconsin, Milwaukee County Medical Complex. She received her BSN from Alverno College and her MSN from Marquette University, Milwaukee, Wisconsin.

Jan Wilson, a nurse clinician in hyperalimentation at Massachusetts General Hospital, Boston, received her BS from St. Joseph's College, Emmitsburg, Maryland.

Laurence W. Wolfe is a clinical pharmacist and adjunct clinical instructor at Temple University Hospital and School of Pharmacy, Philadelphia. He received his BSc in pharmacy at the Philadelphia College of Pharmacy and Science.

ACKNOWLEDGEMENTS
p. 47 Photo courtesy: Moschella, Samuel L., Pillsbury, Donald M., and Hurley, Harry J., *Dermatology,* W. B. Saunders Company, 1975, Volume II, p. 946.
p. 91 Drawing adapted from: Guyton, Arthur C., *Textbook of Medical Physiology,* W. B. Saunders, 1976, p. 52.
p. 100 Photo courtesy: Beyers, Marjorie and Dudas, Susan, *The Clinical Practice of Medical-Surgical Nursing,* Little, Brown and Company, 1977, p. 670. Ron Hurst, photographer.
p. 101 X-ray courtesy: Susan Love Mignogna, RN, ONS, Hahnemann Medical College and Hospital, Philadelphia, Pa.
p. 126 X-rays courtesy: Peter G. Lavine, MD, Crozer-Chester Medical Center, Chester, Pa.
p. 131 EKG courtesy: Peter G. Lavine, MD, Crozer-Chester Medical Center, Chester, Pa.
p. 150 Adapted from: Netter, Frank H., *The Ciba Collection of Medical Illustrations,* 1974, Vol. 5, pp. 94-5.

FOREWORD

There's hardly a disease process or medical intervention that does not involve a threat or a potential threat to a patient's fluid and electrolyte balance. Even patients who are only mildly ill can rapidly develop critical imbalances.

The nurse is the health-care worker who most continually observes and evaluates patients' progress. So the nurse is most logically accountable for assessing and reporting real or potential fluid and electrolyte disturbances.

Very minor changes in a patient's behavior such as slight restlessness, twitching, or a change in breathing patterns may be early signs of imbalance. A knowledgeable nurse can recognize these minor changes, report them accurately, and effectively manage the situation; frequently she can prevent serious or even life-threatening problems.

This Skillbook will help you to build a foundation of competence. It focuses on the *nurse's* role in assessment, record-keeping, and management of fluid and electrolyte disturbances. And it gives real applications of these complex and sometimes difficult-to-grasp principles. This book begins with the physiology of fluids and electrolytes in the balanced state (homeostasis); continues with definitions and tips for recognizing imbalance; describes the function of the key electrolytes and points out what you especially need to remember about them. The most comprehensive section of the book deals with specific clinical situations in which fluid and electrolyte problems dominate. And it describes nursing management in helpful detail. Finally, it reviews treatment techniques, including intravenous therapy, hyperalimentation, and renal and peritoneal dialysis.

Regardless of your nursing practice setting, this Skillbook will give you solid knowledge of fluid and electrolyte disturbances and will make you a more responsive and responsible member of the health-care team.

JOAN DELONG HARRINGTON, RN, BSN, MA
Nephrology Nurse, St. Louis, Missouri
and Coauthor of PATIENT CARE IN RENAL FAILURE

UNDERSTANDING HOMEOSTASIS

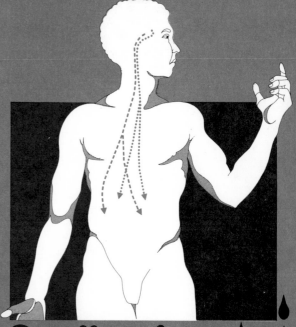

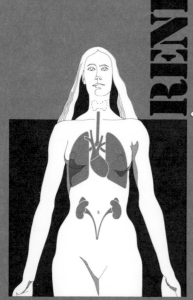

RENIN

feedback

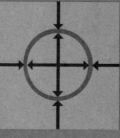

OSMOLALITY

ADH

ISOTONIC

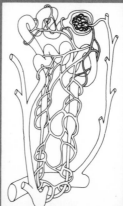

Homeostasis
THE BALANCED STATE

1

BY DIANE DRESSLER, RN, BSN

DO YOU HANG I.V. BOTTLES somewhat mechanically? With the uneasy feeling that you'd rather not think too closely about all those ions and mEqs? If you do, you're not alone or even unusual. Yet, fluid therapy isn't some mysterious alchemy that surpasses understanding. Rather, it's just another treatment technique that, like any other, rests on certain principles and rules. These principles and rules can be understood, and you should understand them.

The internal fluid of the human body works within limited tolerances of volume, acidity, and electrolytes. During illness, this delicate chemical equilibrium is unstable. If it starts to deteriorate, and you don't know what to look for and what to do about it — even before the doctor comes — the patient may get into serious trouble. Knowing what reactions to look for takes a working knowledge of the normal state of chemical balance within the body, what's often called homeostasis.

Fortunately, the nurses who took care of Mrs. Davidson were aware of these homeostatic mechanisms. By correlating her vital signs and her symptoms with laboratory results, they were able to recognize developing imbalance quickly and correct it — before a critical situation could develop.

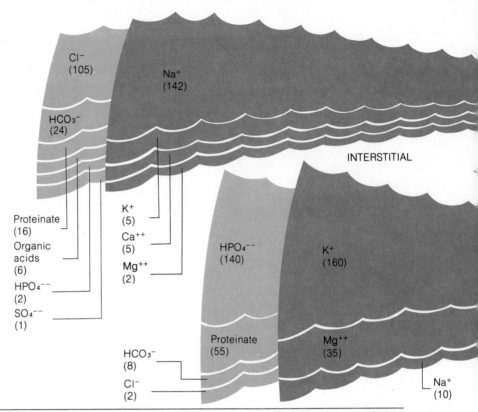

The sea within
As animals evolved from the earliest single-cell organism in the sea and came up on land, they brought their aquatic heritage with them in the form of body fluids. In man these fluids exist in the cells, in the vessels, and between the two, in the interstitial space. The fluids in each compartment contain essential chemicals — electrolytes — in the proportions shown. Together fluids and electrolytes nourish and maintain the body as the sea nourished and maintained the first single-cell organism. They are our heritage from the sea.

Cl^- (105)

Na^+ (142)

HCO_3^- (24)

INTERSTITIAL

Proteinate (16)

Organic acids (6)

HPO_4^{--} (2)

SO_4^{--} (1)

K^+ (5)

Ca^{++} (5)

Mg^{++} (2)

HPO_4^{--} (140)

K^+ (160)

Proteinate (55)

Mg^{++} (35)

HCO_3^- (8)

Cl^- (2)

Na^+ (10)

Mrs. Davidson, a 60-year-old patient receiving radiation therapy, was unable to maintain adequate oral intake because of nausea and vomiting. Consequently she had been receiving a hyperalimentation solution containing 50% dextrose and 8.5% FreAmine plus essential electrolytes and vitamins. On the third day of treatment, her nurses noticed that she seemed lethargic and confused. Her skin was hot and flushed and her mouth dry. Her temperature was 102° F. (38.9° C.). Her blood pressure had decreased from her normal range of 130-140/80-86 to 106/50. Her apical heart rate had increased from 88 to 100. Laboratory data showed a blood sugar of 300 mg/100 ml; a BUN of 40 mg/100 ml, and a serum osmolality of 350 mOsm/kg. Daily weights showed that she had lost 6 lb in 3 days. Her daily urine output was 3200 ml. These signs clearly pointed to dehydration resulting from osmotic diuresis. (Her kidneys were attempting to excrete the excessive glucose.) Nursing interventions emphasized fluid replacement to restore adequate hydration in a person unable to respond to thirst. To correct hyperglycemia, the hyperalimentation solution was temporarily changed to 10% dextrose in water. Mrs. Davidson became much more alert as fluid and electrolyte homeostasis stabilized. Her vital signs and blood sugar level returned to normal.

The complex interplay of chemical changes in Mrs. Davidson's history is typical of patients who are ill. Changes in the volume, distribution, and composition of body fluids can lead to imbalances. The body cannot cope with them, even when fully using its powers of regulation. These changes may come from inadequate intake of essential nutrients, or from structural

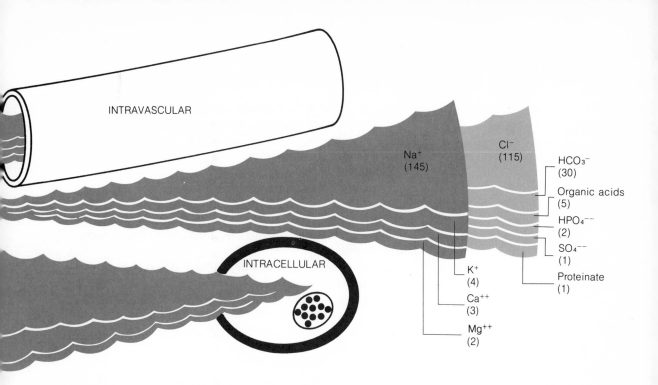

changes due to disease or trauma. As in Mrs. Davidson's case, such imbalances rarely involve simply water or one particular solute. Because of their complex interdependency, a change in one soon leads to a change in another.

We'll discuss the major clinical imbalances in detail in later chapters. But first, let's review the balanced state, what's often called homeostasis, and the regulatory factors that maintain it. Clearly, you need to understand the pattern of fluids and electrolytes as well as you understand the pattern of heart sounds.

The pattern of fluids (volume)

Body fluid — mainly water — accounts for 60% of the total body weight in adults, and 80% in infants. The percentage of total body water varies somewhat with the amount of fat in the body. Since fat is essentially water-free, the leaner the individual, the greater the proportion of water to total body weight. The rest of the body weight is made up of lymph, cell solids, fat, and minerals.

Two main compartments — the intracellular and extracellular — enclose the body fluid. The intracellular compartment is by far the largest, containing the fluid within the 100 trillion cells that make up the human body, and accounts for about 40% of the total body weight. The extracellular compartment contains body fluid in:

- interstitial fluid, in the spaces between cells, which accounts for 15% of total body weight

• plasma, the intravascular fluid within arteries, veins, and capillaries, accounts for 5%. Several other fluid compartments, including the cerebrospinal fluid and intraocular fluid, play a smaller role in fluid and electrolyte balance.

The intracellular compartment contains 25 liters of fluid; the extracellular compartment contains 15 liters including the 5 liters of blood volume. Any change in the amount or composition of these fluids causes serious problems: A 10% fluid loss (about 4 liters) is considered serious; a 20% loss (about 8 liters) is usually fatal.

The fluids in these compartments have different compositions. They are separated by semipermeable membranes, which allow fluids and solutes to move back and forth. Because of this, changes in one compartment produce changes in the others.

Pattern of electrolytes
Body fluids contain two kinds of dissolved substances: those that dissociate in solution (electrolytes) and those that do not. For example, glucose when dissolved in water does not break down into anything smaller. On the other hand, sodium chloride dissociates in solution into sodium cations (+) and chloride anions (−). They are called electrolytes because they will conduct a weak electrical current.

The principal extracellular electrolytes are sodium, calcium, and bicarbonate. The principal cellular electrolytes are potassium, magnesium, and phosphate. Sodium is the dominant extracellular cation; potassium, the dominant *cellular* cation. Chloride is the dominant extracellular anion; phosphate, the dominant *cellular* anion. Each fluid compartment has its own composition of electrolytes, and these must be in the right compartments in the right amounts. The unit of measure used for these electrolytes is the milliequivalent (mEq).

Who's afraid of an mEq?
Why this intimidating term? Why can't we deal with milligrams of potassium or sodium? Because the various electrolytes differ in their *chemical activity* — their capacity to interact with other substances. We use the concept of mEqs which measures electrolytes in terms of their *power,* not their weight. Let's look at a simple analogy. When planning an

elegant dinner party for twelve, you would need to invite 6 men and 6 women, all of whom could converse politely in the same language. It would not help you very much to invite 600 pounds of men and 600 pounds of women.

So, one mEq of any electrolyte has the same chemical combining power as 1 mg of hydrogen. It represents the amount of an electrolyte that will react with a given amount of hydrogen. It expresses the chemical activity of an electrolyte in small whole numbers. And the milliequivalent is more relevant than a unit of weight because one gram of a cation does not necessarily react with one gram of an anion, but one milliequivalent of an anion does. Therefore, the *milliequivalent is the measure of the chemical activity or chemical combining power of an ion.*

In each fluid compartment, the various cations and anions balance each other to achieve electrical neutrality. So, there's no net charge within a fluid compartment. Also keep in mind the great similarity between the two extracellular compartments: blood plasma and interstitial fluids. Although plasma contains a larger amount of protein (which determines colloid osmotic pressure), sodium is the main cation. Chloride and bicarbonate are the main anions in both plasma and interstitial fluid.

Electrolytes profoundly influence water distribution, osmolality, acid/base balance and neuromuscular irritability. For example, the balance of sodium and potassium is essential to homeostasis and is essential for nerve conduction and muscle contraction.

How do water and electrolytes move?

What if the concentration of these ions in either the intra- or extracellular spaces changes? That will cause water to shift from the low concentration to the high concentration space until their concentrations are again equal. This shift shrinks and expands the respective spaces. So, the amount and composition of fluid in each compartment remains relatively stable, but each compartment actually constantly replaces and exchanges ions. A single potassium ion may be in the intravascular compartment one minute, in the interstitial fluid the next minute, and in intracellular fluid the next. All the while, however, the overall potassium content of each compartment remains fairly stable.

You can calculate osmolality
Osmolality is the total number of osmotically active particles per liter of solution. Outside the cells, these particles are mainly sodium and its accompanying anions (chloride and bicarbonate), urea, and glucose. Using routine measurements of sodium and glucose, you can quickly calculate the osmolality of extracellular fluid according to the following formula:

$$osmolality = 2\,[Na\,(mEq/L)] + \frac{10\,[glucose\;mg/100\;ml]}{180}\;(mOsm/kg)$$

Multiply the sodium concentration by 2 to account for the anions that accompany sodium. Multiply the glucose (reported as weight in mg per 100 ml) by 10 to convert it to milligrams per liter. Now divide it by its molecular weight (180) to determine the number of osmotically active particles. Since authorities consider urea a negligible force in osmolality, it is excluded from this calculation.

The normal osmolality of human extracellular fluid ranges between 280 and 294 mOsm/kg.

PERMEABILITY

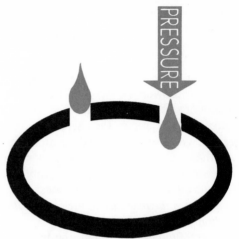

Getting through
Several conditions influence how easily a substance diffuses in body fluid, as shown here. Permeability refers to the size of diffusing particles relative to the size of membrane pores: Smaller particles diffuse more easily.

High pressure intensifies the force under which molecules strike the pores. This force pushes them through the membrane into the area of lower pressure within the cell. Such pressure gradients enable even large molecules to enter the cell.

This changing state is made possible by the semipermeable membranes that separate the fluid compartments. The lipid and protein molecules that make up these membranes are arranged so that only certain substances can pass through them. Pores in these membranes allow the passage of water and small water-soluble substances. Lipid-soluble substances, such as oxygen and carbon dioxide, dissolve in the lipid substances of the membrane. But the semipermeable membrane bars proteins and other intracellular colloids from passing through readily.

Also, certain active metabolic processes at the cell wall exclude certain electrolytes from the cell, while concentrating others within it. How do fluids, electrolytes and other solutes move between cellular and extracellular compartments?

• *By diffusion* — Simple diffusion is the random movement of particles in all directions through a solution or gas. It's what happens when a drop of ink rapidly spreads through a glass of water. In diffusion, molecules spread from an area of greater to lesser concentration. Molecules are in constant motion and tend toward equal concentration in any vessel.

When crossing semipermeable membranes, substances diffuse by:
— passing through the pores, or
— dissolving in the membrane lipid.

But diffusion is not always this simple. Large molecules must pass through membranes by a process called "facilitated diffusion." Sugars, amino acids, and other substances of great molecular size, can diffuse across cell membranes only slowly. They are now thought to cross

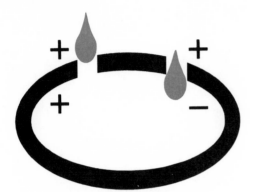

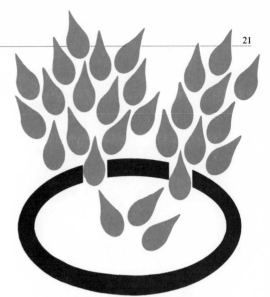

Since opposite charges attract and like charges repel, a difference in electrical charge across a cell membrane facilitates diffusion. For example, positively charged membrane pores are less permeable to the cations sodium and potassium and inhibit their diffusion rate. Because molecules diffuse from an area of high to an area of low concentration in order to achieve equilibrium, the greater the concentration difference across a cell membrane, the more rapid the diffusion rate.

membranes via carrier transport. That is, the material to be diffused combines with certain membrane-bound carrier molecules and crosses the cell membrane as part of a substrate/carrier molecular complex. Apparently, these carrier molecules are confined to the membrane and shuttle back and forth from one side to the other, like ferryboats.

How readily any substance diffuses in body fluid depends on several factors. The first is *permeability.* That depends on the relative size of the membrane pores and the diffusing particles. Obviously, the smallest particles can pass through membrane pores most easily. Water, urea, and chloride are small and diffuse easily; sugars are large and do not. And, since the pores are lined with positively charged ions such as calcium, permeability also depends on the *electrical charge* of the diffusing ion. For example, sodium and potassium have low diffusion rates because they too are positively charged and, so, are repelled by the pores.

Diffusion also depends on: concentration difference, the electrical potential difference, and the pressure difference across the pore. The concentration determines how many molecules strike the outside of a pore each second. So, the greater the *concentration difference,* the greater the diffusion rate. If a *difference in electrical potential* exists across the membrane, diffusion can occur even without a concentration difference. This concept helps explain the transmission of nerve impulses. And finally, *a pressure gradient* influences diffusion. An increase in pressure on one side of the membrane intensifies the molecular forces striking the pores. Pressure gradients explain the movement of substances at the capillary membranes.

• *By osmosis* — Osmosis is water exchange that balances concentration, by which water

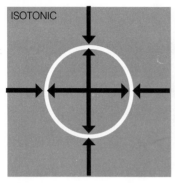

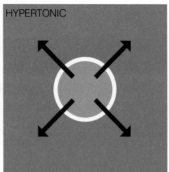

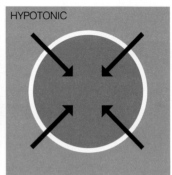

The particulars of concentration
An isotonic fluid has a concentration of dissolved particles, or tonicity, equal to that of the intracellular fluid. When isotonic fluids such as 5% dextrose in water or 0.9% sodium chloride enter the circulation, they cause no net movement of water across the semipermeable cell membrane. And because the osmotic pressure is the same inside and outside the cells, they do not swell or shrink.

A hypertonic fluid has a concentration greater than that of intracellular fluid. When a hypertonic solution such as 3% sodium chloride or 50% dextrose is rapidly infused into the body, water will rush out of the cells to the area of greater concentration and the cells will shrivel. Dehydration can also make extracellular fluid hypertonic, which will lead to the same kind of cellular shrinking.

A hypotonic fluid has a

concentration less than that of intracellular fluid. When a hypotonic solution such as distilled water surrounds a cell, water will diffuse into the intracellular fluid, causing the cell to swell. Inappropriate use of intravenous fluids or severe electrolyte loss will make body fluids hypotonic.
For example, a patient with a sodium deficit after gastric suction may have hypotonic extracellular fluid.

---

moves from a less concentrated solution to a more concentrated one. You probably remember the old axiom, "water goes to salt," which helps you to understand how isotonic, hypotonic, and hypertonic solutions affect body cells. For example, if blood cells are suspended in an *isotonic* solution (one with the same tonicity as plasma — 5% dextrose or 0.9% saline) the osmotic pressure will be the same inside and outside the cell. Therefore, water will not leave or enter the cell, and the shape of the cell will remain the same. If blood cells are placed in a *hypotonic* solution, one less concentrated than the contents of the cell, water will flow into the cells until they swell and burst. Finally, if blood cells are suspended in a *hypertonic* solution, water will move out of the cells until they shrink like raisins.

This brings us to another important term — *osmolality*.

Let's review what osmolality actually means. If a solute is added to water, the amount of water in that solution will be reduced (the solution now contains fewer water molecules per unit volume because some space is taken up by solute molecules). Furthermore, the presence of the solute molecules changes the chemical behavior of water so that, for example, diffusion occurs more slowly. And the boiling and freezing points change. Thus, osmolality measures the *number* of particles in a solution which reduce the concentration and therefore change the chemical potential of body water. You can think of osmolality as the "specific gravity" of body fluids. It is expressed as the number of dissolved particles per unit of water. The unit of

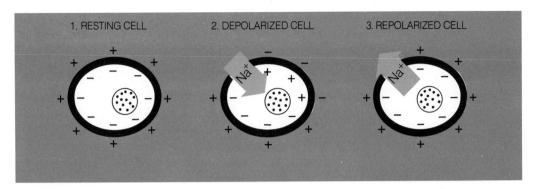

1. RESTING CELL   2. DEPOLARIZED CELL   3. REPOLARIZED CELL

Balancing act
The electrolytes sodium and potassium play a crucial role in neuromuscular functioning through the process of depolarization and repolarization.

In the resting cell (Figure 1), anions accumulate along the inner surface of the cell membrane as cations accumulate along the outer. Stimuli — such as heat, cold, electricity, mechanical damage, or any other factor that temporarily disrupts the normal resting state — cause the cell membrane to become very permeable to sodium. Sodium rushes into the cell, reversing the original resting potential and potassium moves out. This shift is called depolarization (Figure 2).

Within a few milliseconds sodium moves out of the cell again and potassium returns to its cellular compartment. This shift is called repolarization (Figure 3). Repolarization returns the cell to its electrical resting potential.

This electrolyte exchange is transmitted along the axon, causing nerve conduction and muscle contraction. An electrolyte imbalance will affect the synchronization of neuromuscular function, which can lead to irritability of muscles, nerves, and heart. If the nerve stimulus is transmitted during the refractory period of the muscle, there'll be no contraction. If the contraction is sustained, tetany may result.

---

measure is the milliosmole (mOsm). What you need to remember about osmolality:
- The normal osmolality of body fluids is 280-294 mOsm/kg.
- The intracellular and extracellular osmolalities are always equal, and their measurement tells us about overall body hydration, or how concentrated the body fluids are.
- Water diffuses from low osmolality to high osmolality.
- Intracellular fluid rapidly reflects extracellular imbalances because of osmotic equilibrium.
- *By active transport* — The third mechanism for moving fluids and electrolytes is active transport, the force used when the cell membranes must move molecules "uphill" against a concentration gradient. This mechanism uses energy in the form of adenosine triphosphate (ATP) and a carrier substance to transport sodium, potassium, chloride, sugars, and amino acids. It's similar to facilitated diffusion except that it acts against a concentration gradient. The most important example of active transport is the "sodium pump" (or "cation pump") which maintains conduction and contraction in nerve and muscle cells (see insert, p. 91, sodium pump).

Electrolyte imbalances can profoundly affect membrane excitability and normal neuromuscular conduction. You know, for example, that hypocalcemia can lead to uncontrollable depolarization of nerve and muscle cells and hypocalcemic tetany. And hypokalemia decreases neuromuscular excitability, causing muscle weakness or paralysis.

The ins and outs
In a healthy person, the fluids he ingests balance the fluids he excretes (see illustration, opposite page). Water loss via the skin and lungs will increase with increased respiratory rate, fever, a hot dry environment, or injury to the skin such as burns. Water loss via the kidneys varies largely with the amount of solute excreted and with the level of antidiuretic hormone (ADH), which controls the kidneys' reabsorption of water.

● *By filtration* — Transfer of water and dissolved substances through a permeable membrane from a region of high pressure to low pressure is called *filtration*. The force behind filtration is hydrostatic pressure (or capillary pressure), produced by the pumping action of the heart. Examples of filtration include the passage of water and electrolytes from the arterial end of the capillary beds to the interstitial fluid and from the glomerular capillaries of the kidneys into the tubules. Opposing hydrostatic pressure, which tends to force water and electrolytes out of the capillaries, is the plasma colloid osmotic pressure of the plasma proteins, which tends to hold them back.

What do you need to remember about plasma colloid osmotic pressure? The selective retention of colloids such as albumin and globulin in the plasma lowers the concentration of water and electrolytes. The resulting interaction of plasma albumin concentration, capillary hydrostatic blood pressure, and capillary permeability to albumin (collectively called Starling's Law) determine how extracellular fluid moves between the intravascular and interstitial compartments.

What regulates fluids?
The lungs and skin are important monitors of fluid and electrolyte balance. Normally, significant amounts of water and negligible amounts of electrolytes escape through the skin as insensible perspiration and from the lungs in the breath. These insensible losses are considerably higher during fever or in a hot environment. You must consider them for accurate fluid balance measurements.

But the kidneys are the *main* monitors of fluid balance. They control extracellular fluid by regulating:
● concentration of specific electrolytes
● osmolality of body fluids
● volume of extracellular fluid
● blood volume, and
● blood pH.

Kidney function is delicately controlled by hormones and other coordinating mechanisms:
● The *heart and blood vessels* make possible the kidneys' regulatory function by perfusing them with plasma, which must reach the kidneys in sufficient volume.
● The *pituitary* releases a water-saving secretion known as antidiuretic hormone (ADH). ADH causes the kidney tubules

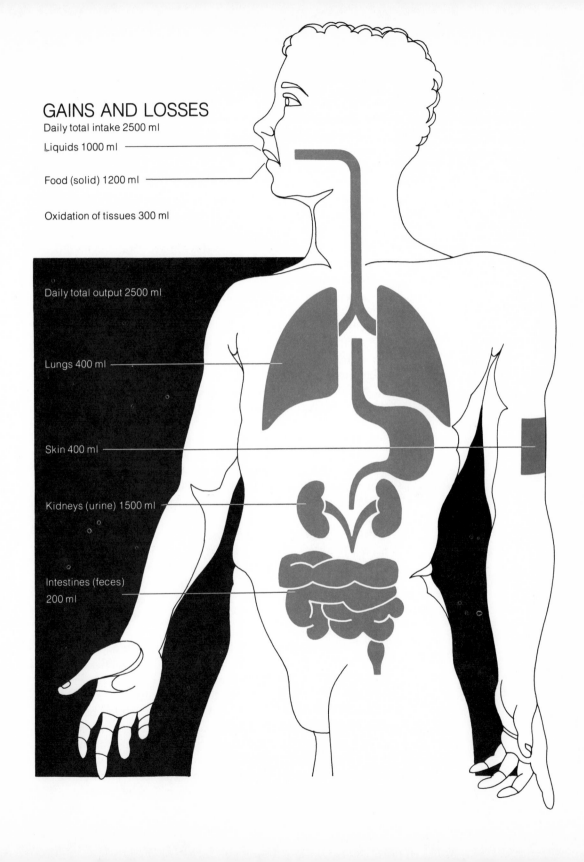

GAINS AND LOSSES
Daily total intake 2500 ml

Liquids 1000 ml

Food (solid) 1200 ml

Oxidation of tissues 300 ml

Daily total output 2500 ml

Lungs 400 ml

Skin 400 ml

Kidneys (urine) 1500 ml

Intestines (feces)
200 ml

At the controls

Many organs control the body's homeostasis as shown on the opposite page: The *pituitary gland* controls secretion of antidiuretic hormone, renal filtration and plasma flow, and adrenal function. The *parathyroids* maintain the level of ionized calcium in the blood and regulate the kidneys' conservation of magnesium. The *lungs* govern the exhalation or retention of carbon dioxide which influences the body's acid-base balance. The *heart and vascular system* nourish the *kidneys* which through filtration, reabsorption and excretion, control the necessary balance of fluids and electrolytes. The *adrenal glands* secrete aldosterone which affects the retention or excretion of sodium, potassium, and water.

to reabsorb more water from the distal renal tubule and collecting duct, thereby making the urine more concentrated. The pituitary gland releases more ADH when increased osmolality of extracellular fluid stimulates the neurohypophysis. Also, anterior pituitary growth hormone helps maintain glomerular filtration, renal plasma flow, and tubular function.

• *Adrenal cortical hormones* normally conserve sodium and chloride, excrete potassium, and enhance water reabsorption in the distal tubules. They do this chiefly via the mineralocorticoid, aldosterone. Aldosterone acts on the kidney tubules to increase the reabsorption of sodium (and along with it, water) and decrease the reabsorption of potassium. The adrenal cortex secretes more aldosterone whenever: extracellular potassium increases; extracellular sodium decreases; or cardiac output drops. Remember, stress tends to cause the kidneys to retain sodium and excrete potassium, resulting in many of the electrolyte imbalances we see in patients.

• *Thirst* regulates fluid intake. Increased osmolality stimulates osmoreceptors in the hypothalamus to give the sensation of thirst.

Thus, depending on circumstances, the kidneys selectively either rid the body of extra water and electrolytes or conserve and return them to the circulation. This explains why infusions of water and electrolytes are useful. The kidneys retain the needed amounts of water and electrolyte and excrete the rest.

Pattern of pH

As you know, pH is a scale from 1 to 15 that chemists use to describe the acidity or alkalinity of a solution, in this case blood. The pH of a fluid tells us its hydrogen ion concentration. Normally the pH of blood is maintained between 7.35 and 7.45. A variation of only 0.4 of a pH unit in either direction can be fatal.

The body regulates its pH through three mechanisms:

• *Blood buffers* neutralize excess acids or alkalis that form as a result of metabolic processes. In plasma, pH is determined by the ratio of bicarbonate to carbonic acid — the principal buffer pair. The ratio of carbonic acid to base bicarbonate is usually 1:20, but this ratio changes as one shifts into the other to help offset changes in hydrogen ion concentration.

• *The lungs* act within minutes to regulate the volatile carbonic acid in the blood through exhalation or retention of

CONTROLLING
ORGANS

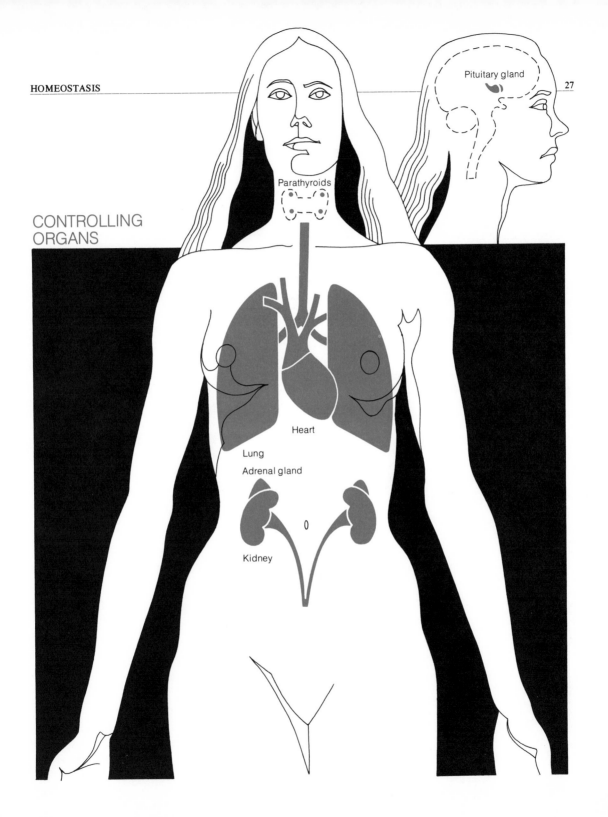

Pituitary gland

Parathyroids

Heart

Lung

Adrenal gland

Kidney

carbon dioxide. If there is an excess of H^+ and the blood is too acidic, the patient may hyperventilate to get rid of excess acid. If there is an inadequate amount of H^+ and blood is too alkaline, the patient may hypoventilate to store CO_2 (carbonic acid) and restore the pH to normal.

• *The kidneys* take hours or days to play their part in acid-base regulation, but they secrete or retain hydrogen or bicarbonate ions until the pH balance is exactly normal.

Remember that you cannot effectively evaluate serum electrolytes without knowing the blood pH. This is true because changes in pH greatly affect the movement of electrolytes across the cell membrane and cause dramatic changes in the serum levels.

Even if you don't use them regularly, review these principles of fluid and electrolyte balance. They regulate the solutes and concentrations of body fluid both inside and outside the cell. Knowing them will help you recognize and correctly cope with deviations from the normal pattern. And such deviations can cause severe illness or even death.

Two Hormones
REGULATORS OF FLUID BALANCE

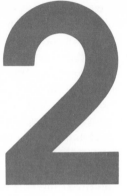

BY JANE LANCOUR, RN, BSN, MSN

UNLESS YOU SPECIALIZE in nursing care of patients with renal disease, you probably haven't thought much about anti-diuretic hormone (ADH) and aldosterone — two of the body's hormonal regulators of fluid excretion. Maybe you haven't thought about them at all since the last time you saw a patient with diabetes insipidus. But you should. Both ADH and aldosterone are now recognized as having far-reaching clinical implications that you're sure to meet sometime or other. For example, ADH is now known to be an important factor in surgical patients and, in fact, in all patients under stress.

What is ADH?
ADH (often called vasopressin) is a polypeptide consisting of eight amino acids. It gets released from the posterior pituitary gland. ADH has an affinity for the renal tubules where it causes reabsorption of water back into the circulation.

ADH causes large quantities of water to be reabsorbed in response to increased osmolality (deficiency of water). In response to decreased osmolality (an excess of water), decreased secretion of ADH allows increased excretion of water to maintain homeostasis. Another hormone, aldosterone,

Hormones for homeostasis
Two main hormones affect the
balance of water and sodium in
the body. The hypothalamus
releases antidiuretic hormone
(ADH) (see opposite page). ADH
acts on the distal renal tubules
and the collecting duct of the
kidney to retain or secrete water.
   Midbrain volume receptors,
sensitive to the serum sodium
load, stimulate the adrenal gland
to release aldosterone.
Aldosterone controls the retention
or secretion of sodium.

causes the renal tubules to retain sodium and water.

Clearly, normal release of ADH and aldosterone rests on an
intricate hormonal system. Interference with any of the links
in this hormonal chain can profoundly affect fluid balance. In
fact, serious fluid imbalance *does* usually follow increased or
decreased release of ADH or aldosterone. But, if you know
what conditions influence their secretion, you can keep ahead
of potential imbalance and take appropriate steps to prevent or
minimize it. Expect increased secretion of ADH:

• *when plasma osmolality is high* (normal is 280 to 294
mOsm/kg): Watch for high osmolality in patients with dehydration or elevations of serum sodium concentration (over 148
mEq/L, serum glucose, or blood urea nitrogen (BUN). High
osmolality stimulates release of ADH, which tries to dilute the
solutes and lower the plasma osmolality toward normal. When
this happens, expect urinary output to fall as low as 400 ml per
day while the urine specific gravity markedly rises.

• *when circulating volume is low:* Stretch receptors in the
atria and blood vessels react to hypovolemia. They stimulate
ADH secretion via a vagal-hypothalamic-hypophyseal path.
This compensatory mechanism increases reabsorption of
water to increase circulating blood volume. Another
mechanism influences hypovolemia in response to low blood
pressure. Baroreceptors in the blood vessels react to low
blood pressure by stimulating ADH release. You may recall
that ADH is a potent vasoconstrictor (as implied by its alter-
nate name, "vasopressin") and markedly increases peripheral
resistance by constricting the arterioles.

• *when the patient suffers pain, unpleasant emotion, or
stress:* Any of these can stimulate ADH production in spite of
hypotonicity (low osmolality). Keep this in mind when caring
for surgical or traumatized patients. Such patients can secrete
ADH even after plasma osmolality is below normal, and therefore easily retain water and become water-toxic.

• *when the patient uses certain drugs and other chemicals:*
Morphine and some anesthetics directly stimulate ADH. So,
in most surgical patients, you must deal with each of those two
potent stimulants for ADH secretion, even without taking into
consideration pain and emotional stress. You must precisely
monitor water and electrolyte balance in surgical patients.

Two other medications, oxytocin (Pitocin) and chlorpropamide (Diabinese), also stimulate ADH production. Ox-

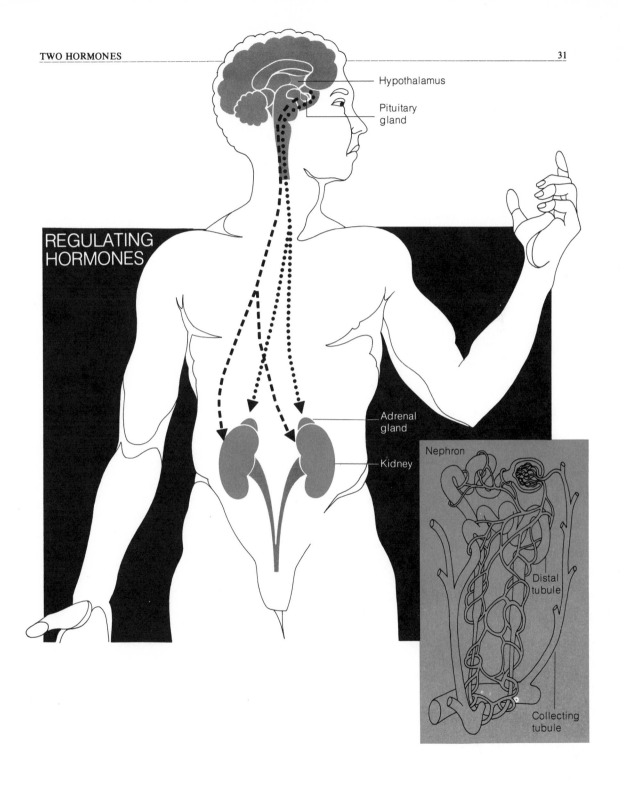

REGULATING
HORMONES

Hypothalamus

Pituitary
gland

Adrenal
gland

Kidney

Nephron

Distal
tubule

Collecting
tubule

ytocin causes water retention in some obstetrical patients probably by directly stimulating the neurohypophysis. Chlorpropamide, an oral hypoglycemic, augments the renal tubular response to circulating ADH, intensifying its effect and producing water retention and hyponatremia (hypotonicity).

• *when the patient receives positive-pressure breathing:* Positive pressure breathing stimulates ADH via the same stretch receptors that react to hypovolemia. So when you see a surgical or trauma patient who has been the victim of stress, has pain, has received morphine and is also receiving positive pressure ventilation, you can consider serious water imbalance almost a certainty. Monitor such a patient's fluid status with particular zeal.

What inhibits ADH?

Increased plasma osmolality, decreased circulating volume, and positive pressure breathing stimulate ADH production. So the opposite conditions — decreased osmolality, increased circulating volume, and negative pressure breathing *inhibit* it. So can alcohol, which explains the marked diuresis that occurs during an alcoholic bout.

Inappropriate ADH a problem

Excessive ADH secretion *despite* normal serum osmolality is called syndrome of inappropriate ADH (SIADH). It can be transient (after trauma, surgery, or stress) or sustained (associated with central nervous system [CNS] disorders, cerebrovascular accident [CVA], pulmonary disorders, and certain lung tumors). For example, intracranial lesions can cause hypersecretion of ADH by directly irritating the supraoptic nuclei. Oat cell lung tumors can themselves secrete ADH, or may stimulate ADH secretion by irritating certain sensory nerves. Certain other conditions (hypothyroidism and some organic intracranial diseases) cause excessive excretion of ADH via an abnormally low "set-point" for osmolality. In these conditions, osmoreceptors react at a lower threshold and trigger ADH secretion even at low osmotic concentrations. Watch for the following characteristic changes that develop in patients with inappropriate secretion of antidiuretic hormone (SIADH):

• low serum sodium
• low urine output (400 to 500 ml/day)

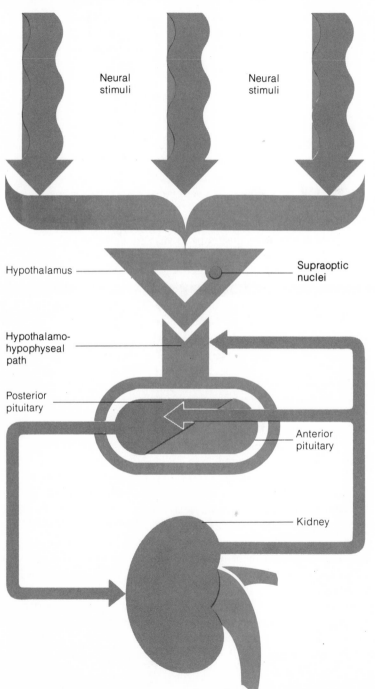

Neural stimuli

Neural stimuli

Hypothalamus

Supraoptic nuclei

Hypothalamo-
hypophyseal
path

Posterior
pituitary

Anterior
pituitary

Kidney

The negative feedback mechanism

When the body produces a hormone vital to homeostasis, what prevents oversecretion? A negative feedback mechanism, one example of which works like this.

Neural impulses from the brain stimulate the supraoptic nuclei in the hypothalamus which forms antidiuretic hormone (ADH). The supraoptic nuclei send ADH via the hypothalamo-hypophyseal tract to the posterior pituitary to be stored and released as needed to the kidneys. The retention of enough water inhibits the posterior pituitary and the hypothalamo-hypophyseal tract from producing and carrying more ADH.

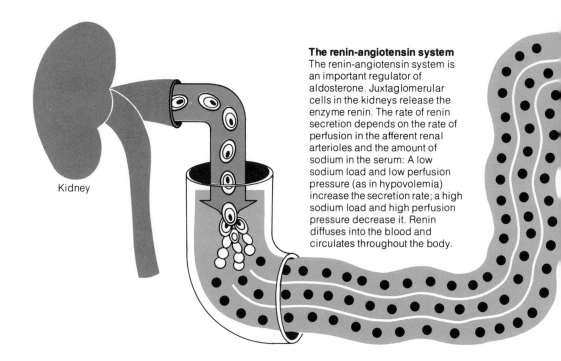

Kidney

The renin-angiotensin system
The renin-angiotensin system is an important regulator of aldosterone. Juxtaglomerular cells in the kidneys release the enzyme renin. The rate of renin secretion depends on the rate of perfusion in the afferent renal arterioles and the amount of sodium in the serum: A low sodium load and low perfusion pressure (as in hypovolemia) increase the secretion rate; a high sodium load and high perfusion pressure decrease it. Renin diffuses into the blood and circulates throughout the body.

- high urine specific gravity
- serum osmolality below 280 mOsm/kg water
- positive water balance (intake exceeds output)
- weight gain
- neurologic symptoms (restlessness, irritability, convulsions, and unresponsiveness).

When ADH is low
If a patient with low ADH secretion can satisfy his thirst sufficiently to replace the fluids lost, he can probably maintain water balance. But he will develop fluid imbalance if his thirst mechanism is impaired; if he has marked dryness of the mouth from nasal oxygen; if he is a mouth breather; if he has an accumulation of oral secretions; or, if he is so incapacitated that he cannot satisfy his thirst. His intake will not balance an excessive output, so he will become severely dehydrated and may go into shock.

As you know, *diabetes insipidus* is one such condition of low circulating ADH. It may have a central or renal cause. Central diabetes insipidus may result from a lesion in the supraoptic nuclei or from head trauma. Or it may follow hypophysectomy or other neurological surgery. And, it may result from renal inability to respond to ADH (which can be congenital, acquired, or iatrogenic).

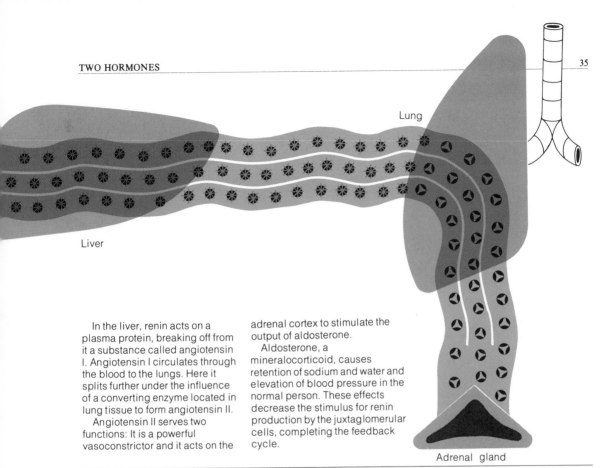

Lung

Liver

In the liver, renin acts on a plasma protein, breaking off from it a substance called angiotensin I. Angiotensin I circulates through the blood to the lungs. Here it splits further under the influence of a converting enzyme located in lung tissue to form angiotensin II.

Angiotensin II serves two functions: It is a powerful vasoconstrictor and it acts on the adrenal cortex to stimulate the output of aldosterone.

Aldosterone, a mineralocorticoid, causes retention of sodium and water and elevation of blood pressure in the normal person. These effects decrease the stimulus for renin production by the juxtaglomerular cells, completing the feedback cycle.

Adrenal gland

You're sure to hear more about one growing iatrogenic cause. This is lithium (Lithane), which is used for treating manic-depressive psychosis. Because lithium strongly interferes with the synthesis, storage, and release of ADH, patients who take it experience excessive thirst and polyuria. If their water intake is inadequate, they may develop marked derangements of fluid and electrolyte balance. You need to keep lithium in mind because its use is becoming quite common. And, patients who need lithium and who undergo major surgery are likely to receive it immediately postoperatively, to maintain their therapeutic blood level. So, when caring for surgical patients who take lithium, add its potential effects on ADH to all the other adverse effects that stress and the surgery itself can provoke. Watch for the following signs of diabetes insipidus:

- high urinary output (15 to 16 L/day)
- low specific gravity (1.000 to 1.005)
- excessive thirst (if the patient is responsive)
- fair to poor skin turgor
- dry mucous membranes
- negative fluid balance (output exceeds intake).

If diabetes insipidus is permanent, it requires treatment with vasopressin tannate in oil (Pitressin Tannate). Remember to shake the bottle of Pitressin well before filling the syringe because the active ingredient tends to settle on the bottom. A single dose is given *deep* I.M. and is not repeated until polydipsia and polyuria reoccur. If the diabetes insipidus is transient, the only treatment is to provide enough water intake to balance output.

How to assess ADH for imbalance? Several things you must do make it easier:

• *Record intake and output accurately.* If intake exceeds output, fluid balance is positive; if output exceeds intake, fluid balance is negative. Average urinary output is 1500 ml/day.

• *Weigh the patient daily at the same time, with the same kind of clothing and with the same scale.* (Body weight is the best measure of fluid status.)

• *Determine urine specific gravity.* Low specific gravity means dilute urine; high specific gravity, concentrated urine.

• *Watch for thirst.* Remember the special situations that can interfere with thirst or with the patient's capacity to respond to it: aphasia, old age, unconsciousness, confusion, dependency, tracheostomy or use of respirator.

• *Provide excellent oral hygiene at least three times daily.* This encourages normal taste and thirst perception.

Aldosterone, the other regulator

Aldosterone is a mineralocorticoid secreted by the adrenal cortex in response to certain stimuli. Aldosterone influences the renal tubules to increase their reabsorption of sodium in exchange for excreting potassium.

What stimulates aldosterone release?

• *High serum potassium levels* elicit aldosterone release through a potent feedback system. A rise of less than 2 mEq/L can *triple* the secretion of aldosterone. Obviously, without a functioning aldosterone system, man could easily die of hypo- or hyperkalemia.

• *Hyponatremia,* which can follow sodium restriction or prolonged diuresis, stimulates the adrenal cortex to secrete more aldosterone. This promotes reabsorption of sodium from the renal tubules.

• *Hypovolemia* stimulates secretion of renin which elicits aldosterone secretion. Hypovolemia elicits aldosterone secretion even in patients who simultaneously have edema or ascites, further complicating their already severe imbalance.

• *The renin-angiotensin system* is another important regulator of aldosterone. Certain conditions (upright posture, low-salt diet, dehydration, hemorrhage, and hypotension) that decrease the perfusion pressure in the afferent renal arterioles provoke renin release from the juxtaglomerular cells. Renin release starts a compensatory chain of events which includes secretion of aldosterone and ends with *increased* arteriolar pressure and *decreased* renin secretion.

When aldosterone secretion rises, you can expect certain clinical problems. *Hypokalemia* is especially likely. Aldosterone causes marked potassium excretion in exchange for sodium reabsorption. (As the sodium is reabsorbed, it causes electronegativity in the renal tubules; this electrical gradient attracts the potassium into the kidney tubule, promoting its excretion.)

Also, *alkalosis* can occur. As sodium gets reabsorbed it causes hydrogen to be secreted into the kidney tubules — also as a result of rising electronegativity in the tubules. For each hydrogen ion secreted, a bicarbonate ion enters the body fluid which shifts the hydrogen ion concentration toward alkalosis. Normally, this increased pH is compensated by the normal acid-base regulatory mechanism over a period of a few days.

And finally, *hypertension* may follow increased aldosterone secretion. Some patients who use oral contraceptives develop hypertension along with hypokalemia. This is attributed to estrogen which raises the renin levels (renin-angiotensin system). Investigators have found that renal transplant patients who receive steroids retain sodium and tend to be hypertensive. They also found that steroids are actually *converted* to aldosterone producing a four-fold rise of aldosterone over normal levels. Such patients have been treated successfully with spironolactone (Aldactone).

Knowing what stimulates aldosterone release, you would expect the following opposing situations to inhibit it.

• *Hypernatremia or hypokalemia* elicit a negative feedback response that holds back aldosterone in an effort to maintain electrolyte balance.

• *Spironolactone* (a diuretic) directly antagonizes aldosterone and therefore conserves potassium. So, when caring for patients who are taking spironolactone, watch for hyperkalemia.

Conversely, when aldosterone secretion falls, you can expect the opposite clinical problems — hyperkalemia and acidosis. If aldosterone is unavailable to facilitate reabsorption of sodium, potassium gets absorbed instead. As the potassium is reabsorbed, so is hydrogen. This produces metabolic acidosis. Also look for *decreased cardiac output*. When decreased sodium and water reabsorption reduce the extracellular fluid volume, they also reduce the venous return to the right atrium. With preload thus decreased, less volume is available with each stroke, and cardiac output falls.

How to identify aldosterone imbalances?

- Monitor laboratory data for high or low potassium levels.
- Watch for symptoms of potassium imbalance.
- Watch for hypertension associated with hypokalemia.
- Monitor pH on laboratory reports.
- Look for signs of diminished cardiac output: decreased CVP; thready pulse; hypotension; and diminished urinary output.
- Accurately record intake and output
  — evaluate for positive or negative fluid balance
  — record weight daily
  — watch for increased thirst.
- Report abnormal findings promptly.

SKILLCHECK 1

1. Sarah Friedman, a 64-year-old librarian, was hospitalized with the diagnosis of a lung mass. An extensive diagnostic work-up, which included an open-lung biopsy, confirmed a diagnosis of oat-cell carcinoma. During her evaluation for radiation therapy, you noticed a change in her urine output. For the past 2 days, her urinary output was only 420 ml/day and 500 ml/day despite adequate intake. She has also gained 4 lbs over the past 3 days. The lab reported her last serum sodium at 121 mEq/L. What do you suspect might be the problem?

2. Which of these fluid compartments is the most susceptible to loss of fluid? The intracellular or extracellular compartment?

3. How does atherosclerotic deterioration contribute to the elderly person's extreme susceptibility to dehydration?

4. Jerry Miller is a 42-year-old alcohol-abuser admitted to your unit with cirrhosis of the liver. You learn from his history that this is a chronic problem, and he has been admitted before with hepatic decompensation. Although he's quite slender, Mr. Miller now has +4 pitting edema of both ankles and feet and an enlarged abdomen due to ascites. Among other treatment his doctor has ordered 4 units of albumin. Why?

5. *True or False?* Water content of foods and fluids ingested accounts for all of the body's fluid intake.

6. A urinometer measures the density of a urine specimen. What does this mean?

7. Why are infants especially vulnerable to dehydration?

8. Mr. Gunther George, a 48-year-old accountant with cirrhosis and ascites, was admitted to the emergency room with severe GI bleeding. For 2 days he was in moderate shock with all the classical symptoms: oliguria, hypotension, tachycardia, tachypnea, cool clammy skin, and apathy. He was finally stabilized after numerous whole-blood transfusions and continuous iced saline lavages. Endoscopy revealed gastritis and no gastric ulcer so Mr. George was continued on I.V. therapy and nasogastric suction for several days. In checking him one evening, the nurse noticed that his abdomen looked swollen. Checking further, she found presacral edema and decreased urinary output. His vital signs were stable but he complained of weakness and nausea. The nurse reported these changes to an intern who then ordered I.V. Lasix. The nurse questioned this order. Why? Would Lasix have relieved his symptoms? What is causing his edema?

9. All but one of the following factors increase water and sodium retention by a common mechanism: a) morphine; b) stress; c) hypovolemia; d) positive pressure ventilation; e) oxytocin; f) high plasma osmolality; g) alcohol. What is the common mechanism? Which factor does not belong?

(Answers on page 197)

RECOGNIZING IMBALANCE

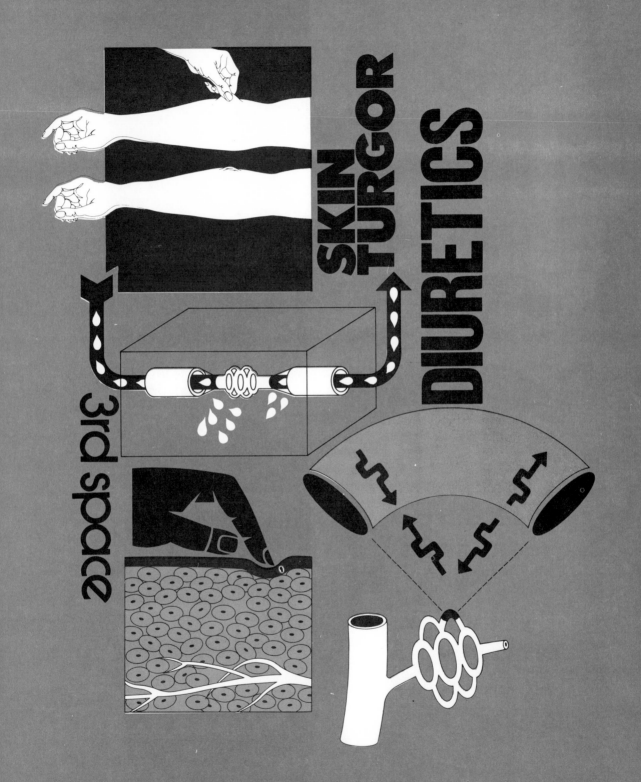

Assessment
HOW TO IMPROVE IT

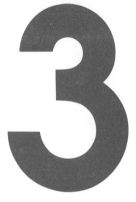

BY ALICE GILLIS, RN, BSN

CAN YOU QUICKLY IDENTIFY the patient who will need intake and output (I and O) records? Do you know when to begin such record keeping on your own? Which patients need electrolyte monitoring? And what their lab results mean? If you don't, your assessment of fluid and electrolyte imbalance is less than it should be.

Most of the data for assessing fluid imbalance are gathered at the bedside and you, the nurse, are mainly responsible for it. No matter how many doctors may attend the patient, you see him the most and are in the best position to notice and evaluate even subtle changes in his condition. Your skills at assessment can make a crucial difference in the patient's treatment. So your data collection begins from the moment the patient enters your care.

Because electrolyte disturbances produce notably non-specific symptoms, they can only be confirmed with laboratory data. For these reasons, your assessment depends on well developed observational skills and an understanding of electrolyte balance. Naturally, intelligent assessment of fluid and electrolyte balance requires a working knowledge of the body fluid compartments, osmosis, osmolality, diffusion, and electrolytes, and how they affect body systems. No less important is an easy familiarity with the terms used for measuring fluid and electrolyte changes — mols, milliequivalents, and such. To make your assessment precise, you need to know what diseases and conditions are most likely to cause imbalance; which patients are most vulnerable to such changes; how to recognize imbalance when it occurs; how to keep meaningful intake and output records; and how to interpret your findings.

Identify patients at risk

First ask yourself — does the patient have any disease or injury that can disrupt body fluid balance? What kind of imbalance usually follows this disease or condition? Is the patient taking any medications or treatment that affects fluid balance (such as steroids or diuretics)?

Know the disease or trauma states that have the greatest potential for altering fluid balance. For example, expect and watch for signs and symptoms of fluid deficit in patients with some kidney diseases, ulcerative colitis, diabetes mellitus, burns, salicylate poisoning (because of hyperventilation), cerebral injuries, diabetes insipidus, and hormonal imbalances (antidiuretic hormone [ADH] and aldosterone). Expect and watch for dehydration when caring for the elderly and for children with febrile infections. Expect and watch for symptoms and signs of fluid overload in patients with congestive heart failure, acute renal insufficiency, cerebral lesions that cause excessive ADH secretion, psychogenic polydipsia, and adrenal insufficiency.

Preventing imbalance is easier if you know what to look for. So learn to anticipate the kind of imbalance that usually accompanies the loss of a specific body fluid. For example...excessive loss of gastric juice often leads to sodium, potassium, magnesium and chloride deficit, and metabolic alkalosis. Excessive perspiration leads to water and sodium deficit. Large losses from open wounds lead to deficit of water, sodium, calcium, and protein. Increased insensible water loss (through lungs and skin) leads to dehydration and increased sodium concentration in the extracellular fluid. The normal amount of such loss ranges from 600 to 1,000 ml daily and is increased by anything that accelerates metabolism. The increase in insensible water loss is roughly 50 to 75 ml per degree of Fahrenheit temperature elevation per 24 hours.

Some Laboratory Tests For Evaluating Fluid Status

LAB TEST	NORMAL VALUE	SIGNIFICANCE
Serum osmolality Measures particles exerting osmotic pull per unit of water; reflects total body hydration	280 to 294 mOsm/kg	• Increases in dehydration. • Decreases with water overload.
BUN (blood urea nitrogen) Reflects difference between rate of urea synthesis and its excretion by the kidneys	10 to 20 mg/100 ml	• Increases with decreased renal blood flow or urine production, dehydration, some neoplasms, and certain antibiotics. • Decreases in pregnancy, overhydration, severe liver disease and malnutrition.
Hematocrit Measures portion of blood volume occupied by RBCs	Female: 37 to 47 ml/100 ml Male: 40 to 54 ml/100 ml	• Increases in dehydration. • Decreases with low RBCs or with normal hemoglobin and water overload.
Creatinine (serum) Measures products of muscle metabolism	0.5 to 1.5 mg/100 ml	• Elevated when 50% or more of the nephrons are destroyed.
Urine osmolality Measures number of particles per unit of water in urine	50 to 1200 mOsm/L (depends upon the circulating titer of ADH and the rate of urinary solute excretion)	• Reflects changes in urine contents more accurately than specific gravity, but depends on the prior state of hydration. It should be 1½ times that of serum.
Urine Specific Gravity (S.G.)	1.010 to 1.030	• Increases with any condition causing hypoperfusion of kidneys leading to oliguria e.g. shock, severe dehydration. • Decreases when renal tubules lose their ability to reabsorb water and concentrate urine as in early pyelonephritis.
Urine pH	4.6 to 8.0 (Average 6.0)	• Increases in metabolic and respiratory alkalosis; in the presence of magnesium ammonium phosphate stones; with certain urea-splitting infections (Pseudomonas, Proteus, E.Coli) • Decreases in the presence of uric acid stones, metabolic and respiratory acidosis. • In renal acidosis, pH may be normal or slightly more acidic only when the plasma HCO_3^- is very low.

Also keep in mind the particular nursing observations that apply to body fluid and electrolyte disturbances. These include: temperature, pulse, respirations, blood pressure, skin and membrane changes, speech changes, fatigue threshold, behavior, skeletal muscle function, anorexia, thirst, and sensory changes. Confirm suspected imbalances with the following data: specific gravity of urine, osmolality, urine volume (intake and output), daily body weights, and blood gases.

Know what vital signs tell
Fever increases metabolism and thus increases fluid loss. It also increases the respiratory rate which promotes loss of water vapor from the lungs. So always report it promptly.

The pulse also offers valuable clues to fluid and electrolyte status. Evaluate the patient's pulse according to rate, volume, regularity, and ease of obliteration. The average rate for adults is 70 to 80 beats per minute but varies with physical conditioning. Increased pulse rate may indicate sodium excess or magnesium deficit; decreased pulse rate, magnesium excess. A weak, irregular, and rapid pulse suggests severe potassium deficit; weak, irregular, slow pulse suggests severe potassium excess. Bounding pulse, not easily obliterated, occurs in volume excess and circulatory overload. Rapid, weak, thready pulse occurs in sodium deficit, interstitial fluid shift, and hypovolemic circulatory collapse.

Respiratory changes point mainly to body pH changes. Evaluate respiration according to rate, depth, and regularity. Expect to see slow, shallow respirations with intermittent periods of apnea in severe metabolic alkalosis. Metabolic acidosis produces the opposite: deep, fast respirations (that may be as fast as 50 respirations per minute).

Clues from veins, skin, and speech
Changes in the *peripheral veins* offer clues to the patient's plasma volume. Normally, elevating the hands causes their veins to empty in 3 to 5 seconds; lowering them causes them to fill again in 3 to 5 seconds. In hypovolemic states (secondary to extracellular fluid deficit or interstitial fluid shift) the hand veins take longer than 3 to 5 seconds to fill. Slow filling of hand veins often precedes hypotension when the patient is in an early stage of shock. When plasma volume is low, the veins are less visible than usual. When plasma volume rises (in

hypervolemia or circulatory overload) the hands take longer than 3 to 5 seconds to *empty*. In that case, the peripheral veins are engorged and highly visible.

Skin turgor tells. Normally, pinched skin falls back to its normal position when released. But in a person with fluid deficit, the skin may remain slightly raised for several seconds. In the elderly, or very thin persons with inelastic skin, this may not be a dependable sign. A dry mouth and lips may be due to fluid deficit or to mouth breathing.

Changes in the pattern, ease, and sound of speech may point to imbalances in fluid, potassium, or calcium. Changes in fatigue patterns often point to potassium imbalance. Also notice the patient's appearance. Drawn look and sunken eyes suggest dehydration; puffy eyelids and fuller cheeks than usual suggest fluid excess.

Know when to measure intake and output

Truly accurate intake and output records are notably difficult to achieve. Yet, they are singularly important to the patient in that they shape the choice of therapy. The doctor is certain to base critical diagnostic and therapeutic judgments on the information they contain.

Many conditions inevitably produce fluid imbalance. Such conditions include burns or other massive injuries, any major surgery, any known or suspected electrolyte imbalance, acute renal failure, oliguria, congestive heart failure, any abnormal body fluid loss, lower nephron nephrosis, and treatment with diuretics, or with adrenocortical steroids. Whenever you care for a patient with any of these conditions, record intake and output even if it has not been ordered. Don't wait for the doctor to request it, for he may assume you will keep such records on your own. So, automatically initiate I and O records in any patient in whom you suspect a real or potential water or electrolyte problem. What should I and O records include? Intake should include all fluids, plus foods liquid at room temperature. Output should include urine, vomitus, diarrhea, drainage and blood. Remind the ambulatory patient whose output you must measure that he must use a bedpan or urinal and *must not* discard his urine until it's measured. Your I and O records should tell the amount and time of day that fluid is taken in or excreted. Note and estimate perspiration. And measure the contents of all drainage bottles.

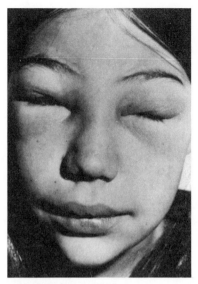

More than the obvious
When assessing for edema, make sure you check more than just arms and legs. Patients with anasarca or renal failure may collect fluid around the eye, as you can see above, or in the sacral area, if they are bedridden. Take time to observe your patient carefully so you can recognize early signs of fluid and electrolyte imbalance.

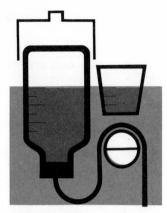

Rule of thumb
Visible fluids (1200 ml), plus three meals (1000 ml), plus water of oxidation (300 ml) should exceed the daily urine output (1500 ml) by at least 500 ml. Minimum urine output in an adult should be 600 ml.

Avoid common sources of error

The possibilities for error in measuring and recording fluid gains or losses seem limitless, but certain errors happen more often than others. Here are some common ones:

• body fluids are discarded or intakes not recorded because some member of the staff did not know which patients needed I and O measurement

• someone failed to explain the need for measuring I and O to the patient, his family, or the dietician.

• putting off to a more convenient time and then forgetting to record a drink of water or an emptied urinal

• guessing amounts instead of measuring fluids

• failure to measure small amounts of fluid accurately (using calibrated cups helps)

• incorrectly estimating fluid taken as ice (remember, a full glass of ice equals a half glass of water when melted)

• assuming that all empty containers of fluid were emptied by the patient (instead of by visitors)

• losing track of infusions from shift to shift

• not estimating perspiration (one necessary bed change represents about 1 liter of fluid lost); or lost vomitus

• failure to: estimate fluid lost in incontinent urine, diarrhea or wound exudate; check the catheter for patency when urine drainage decreases; measure urinary output accurately; and record fluid not returned after irrigation.

Daily body weights essential

Although intake equals output, not all the items are measurable. But a daily body weight can give the best overall picture of the patient's fluid status and it's the easiest record to obtain. Weight loss occurs when the total fluid intake is less than the total fluid output. Remember, however, that loss to the body of effective fluids occurs in interstitial fluid shift. *But such loss,* which can cause a serious fluid volume deficit, *does not change the patient's body weight.* For accurate weight records, be sure to weigh the patient daily, at the same time (usually before breakfast), in the same kind of clothing, and on the same scale. To confirm electrolyte balance, you must rely heavily upon laboratory data (see table). But certain signs and symptoms apparent at the bedside help you to know what tests are needed (see also Chapter 8 to 12.)

Shift To Third Space
WHEN TO EXPECT IT

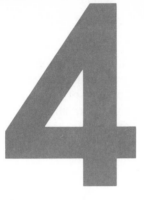

BY MARILYN TWOMBLY, RN, BSN, MSN

YOU KNOW THE SHIFT into third space in its most localized and innocuous form as the familiar blister that follows a small burn...or the swelling in a sprained ankle. At the other extreme, you've seen its generalized and most perilous form in the severely burned patient. Simply defined, "third spacing" is the shift of fluid from the vascular to the interstitial space due to lowered plasma proteins, increased capillary permeability, or lymphatic blockage secondary to trauma, inflammation, or disease. This shift can be localized to a single area or organ. Or it can spread throughout the body. Lately, third space fluid shift has been recognized as a major factor in the fluid balance of patients who've undergone abdominal surgery.

Important fluid and electrolyte changes inevitably occur after repair of an abdominal aneurysm, colon resection, or small-bowel resection. These changes stem mainly from loss of blood and gastric secretions and from intravenous infusions. If the patient's bowel also perforates and he develops peritonitis, the resulting inflammatory response can be enormous and can produce *massive* fluid shift. Despite these massive volumes, "third space" fluid is essentially invisible.

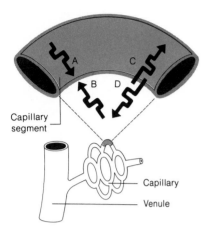

Capillary
segment

Capillary

Venule

Under pressure
Four different pressures move
fluid through the capillary
membrane:
A. *Capillary pressure* is the
pressure fluid within the capillary
exerts outward against the
membrane, like water filling a
balloon;
B. *Interstitial fluid pressure* exerts
a similar pressure inward against
the capillary membrane;
C. *Plasma colloid osmotic
pressure,* a magnet-like attraction
of proteins, pulls fluid from the
interstitial space into the
capillary;
D. *Interstitial fluid colloid osmotic
pressure,* another "protein
magnet" in the opposite direction,
draws fluid from the capillary out
into the third space.

You can see it only indirectly through abdominal distention or
increasing abdominal girth. Where does all this fluid hide?
Much is trapped in the tissue spaces inside the abdomen: the
walls and lumen of the small and large bowel, the omentum,
and the peritoneal covering.

To understand why such unusual fluid shifts happen, you
need to review how fluids move through the capillaries and
lymph system. Four pressures exist at the capillary membrane
which control filtration, reabsorption and, consequently, fluid
equilibrium (see margin). Normally the total outward force at
the arterial end is greater than the total inward force. This
means that about one-tenth of the fluid filtered at the arteriole
is not reabsorbed at the venule. If this were to continue unchecked, the interstitial space would eventually overload with
fluid.

Lymph's crucial role
The lymph system is the accessory route whereby excess
interstitial fluid and leaked proteins — the leftover one-tenth
that cannot get back into the capillary — can eventually flow
back into the vascular space. The terminal lymphatics can
absorb this excess fluid because their special structure readily
accommodates large protein molecules. Without a functioning
lymph system, a person can die within 24 hours.

Normally, the lymph system works efficiently, given small
pressure fluctuations of the interstitial fluid. (Normal interstitial fluid pressure is around minus 7 mm Hg.) Edema will not
develop until something increases this fluid pressure, driving it
above 0 mm Hg. This now-positive pressure exerts a powerful
force on the lymphatics, compressing and collapsing them.
The final result is massively increased tissue fluid volume —
edema.

Expect abnormal fluid pressures in four situations:

• *When capillary pressure is high,* high hydrostatic force
pushes more fluid out of the capillary at the arterial end than is
picked up at the venous end. This extra fluid raises the interstitial fluid pressure. This explains the edema in heart failure.

• *When plasma proteins are low,* capillary pressure (an outward force) overbalances the inward pull of the plasma colloid
osmotic pressure; so fluid flows out but cannot be reabsorbed.
This explains the edema in patients with: inability to make
albumin (liver disease); protein loss (nephrosis or burns);

long-term protein deficit (malnutrition); and protein loss to other compartments (inflammatory response).

• *When the lymph system is blocked,* as in metastatic involvement of the lymph nodes, and after wide resection of tumors and lymph nodes.

• *When the capillaries are too permeable,* plasma proteins escape through the capillary pores, decreasing the plasma colloid osmotic pressure and increasing the tissue colloid osmotic pressure. This pulls fluid out of the vascular space into the tissues. Such fluid shift occurs in septic shock, burns, and allergic reactions. It's a major cause of the hypovolemia that often follows abdominal surgery.

Third spaced fluid occurs in two phases: first loss, then reabsorption. Your nursing goals change somewhat, depending on which phase the patient's in.

First phase: Loss
The loss phase immediately follows surgery or trauma; and depending on the nature and extent of injury, it may last from 48 to 72 hours. During this phase, increased capillary permeability allows protein leakage in areas of inflammation and trauma. This, in turn, shifts fluid from the vascular to the interstitial spaces. During this phase, even if the patient is receiving adequate intravenous fluid replacement, the fluid does not stay in the vascular compartment and the patient may become hypovolemic. Watch for these clinical signs of hypovolemia:
• decreased blood pressure
• increased pulse rate
• low central venous pressure
• decreased urine output
• increased urine specific gravity (because solute content is high compared to volume).

During this phase, the patient's total *intake* of fluid exceeds total *output* of fluid, often by as much as a ratio of 3:1. For example, his intravenous fluid may be replaced at a rate of 125 to 175 ml/hour, while urine output may range from 30 to 70 ml/hour. This reflects a massive leakage of fluid into the tissue spaces where it becomes trapped. Depending on the amount of fluid thus "third-spaced," the patient will show a transient weight gain.

Serum electrolyte levels of sodium, chloride, and potassium

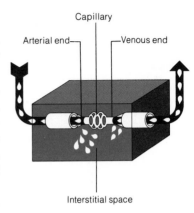

Capillary

Arterial end — — Venous end

Interstitial space

The ends of pressure
The pressure at the arterial end of the capillary is almost three times higher than at the venous end. This pressure differential is an important key to the movement of fluids through the capillary network.

Fluid leaves the capillary bed at the arterial end. It reenters the capillary bed at the venous end through reabsorption. Because the net outward force is greater than the net inward force, 10% of the fluid filtered at the arterial end is not reabsorbed at the venous end. If this continued unchecked, the interstitial space would eventually be overloaded with fluid.

But the lymph system picks up this remaining 10% along with certain proteins and other large molecules too big to reenter the capillary, and returns them to the heart.

The game fluid plays

When extracellular fluid accumulates and becomes trapped in the interstitial space, the body cannot readily transport it back into the circulation. It remains there, in what is called the third space, physiologically useless.

Several disorders cause fluid to shift into the third space, as you can see in our Fluid Shift Game on the opposite page. It's designed to illustrate the movement of body fluid between the vascular, interstitial, and lymph compartments.

may vary, depending on the kind and quantity of fluids infused. If sodium and chloride have been inadequately replaced but fluid volume is high, expect low serum sodium and chloride levels to reflect a dilutional effect. Conversely, if these electrolytes have been replaced, but fluid volume is inadequate, expect laboratory values to show hemoconcentration: higher hematocrit, hemoglobin, sodium, and chloride values.

Extremely important during this phase: Replace the lost plasma proteins by giving albumin or plasmanate. Such replacement increases the plasma colloid osmotic pressure and prevents fluid loss from the capillary, and it may promote reabsorption of excess fluid in the tissue spaces. In most severe injuries, even adequate colloid replacement cannot totally prevent interstitial shift. But it can control and keep it to a minimum. A helpful technique in managing colloid replacement is to give a diuretic immediately after the colloid infusion. This will pull tissue fluid into the vascular space and then immediately allow the kidneys to excrete it.

Two major goals

During the phase of fluid loss to the third space, your nursing interventions have two important objectives: prevent hypovolemia and renal failure. To prevent hypovolemia, you need to monitor blood pressure, pulse, central venous pressure, urine output, and urine specific gravity frequently. Report changes immediately. Be precise about the kind and amount, when giving intravenous fluid replacement. Replace vascular colloid as ordered, and *as soon as it is ordered.* When diuretics follow colloid replacement, remember to carefully monitor potassium levels.

To prevent renal failure, you need to carefully and continuously monitor kidney function. For example, expect the urine specific gravity to be high, except during diuresis. Watch for a rise in creatinine and blood urea nitrogen (BUN) values, for they may signal early renal deterioration. Keep in mind that the *quantity* of urine reflects vascular volume; the *quality* reflects kidney function. Be sure to keep accurate records of intake and output. To do this, weigh the patient daily in the same kind of clothes, under the same conditions, at the same time (i.e. before breakfast), and with the same scale.

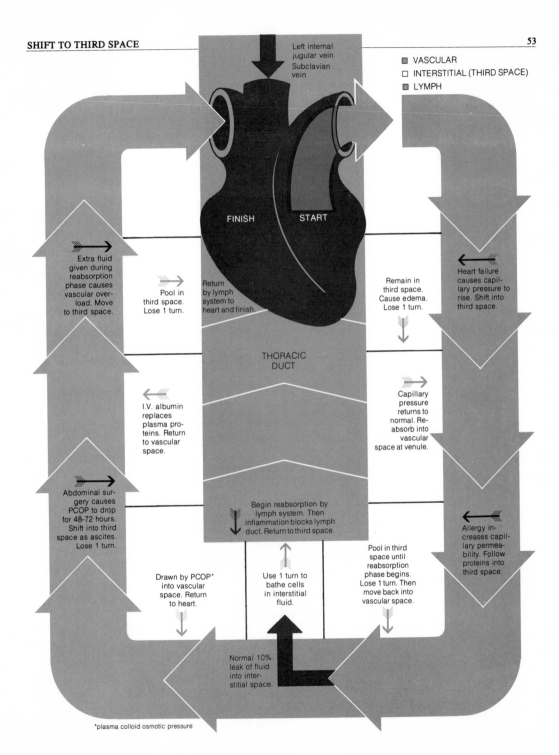

VASCULAR
INTERSTITIAL (THIRD SPACE)
LYMPH

Left internal jugular vein
Subclavian vein

FINISH START

THORACIC DUCT

Extra fluid given during reabsorption phase causes vascular overload. Move to third space.

Pool in third space. Lose 1 turn.

Return by lymph system to heart and finish.

Remain in third space. Cause edema. Lose 1 turn.

Heart failure causes capillary pressure to rise. Shift into third space.

I.V. albumin replaces plasma proteins. Return to vascular space.

Capillary pressure returns to normal. Reabsorb into vascular space at venule.

Abdominal surgery causes PCOP to drop for 48-72 hours. Shift into third space as ascites. Lose 1 turn.

Begin reabsorption by lymph system. Then inflammation blocks lymph duct. Return to third space.

Pool in third space until reabsorption phase begins. Lose 1 turn. Then move back into vascular space.

Allergy increases capillary permeability. Follow proteins into third space.

Drawn by PCOP* into vascular space. Return to heart.

Use 1 turn to bathe cells in interstitial fluid.

Normal 10% leak of fluid into interstitial space.

*plasma colloid osmotic pressure

Second phase: Reabsorption

Once trauma and inflammation subside, the fluid in the tissue spaces begins to be reabsorbed. As injured tissues heal, capillaries repair themselves and normal permeability returns; lymphatic blockage decreases as new channels form and old ones heal. Finally, plasma protein levels return to normal via replacement and reabsorption from tissues. This, in turn, normalizes capillary pressures and, therefore, restores normal capillary fluid filtration and reabsorption.

During this phase, the extra fluid volume formerly held in the tissue spaces shifts back into the vascular compartment and is excreted through the kidneys. Vascular volume rises transiently. In most cases, this normalizing process takes place rather easily. But you need to be aware of it because of the need to limit the amount of external replacement at the time of this internal shift. Extra fluid given at this time can cause vascular overload with increased blood pressure, rapid pulse rate, and steadily rising central venous pressure. So, decrease intravenous replacement at this time, especially if the patient is beginning to take oral fluids.

You can recognize the onset of the reabsorption phase by an increase in urine output that's often quite dramatic. Hourly outputs may range as high as 200 ml per hour. During this phase, expect the specific gravity and electrolyte values to be low due to the dilutional effect of the increased vascular fluid volume. Total fluid output will exceed total fluid intake by as much as three to one. And the patient will show a weight loss, often to preoperative or pre-trauma weight.

At all times during this phase, you need to watch carefully for signs of circulatory overload. Monitor vital sign changes. Watch especially for increased central venous pressure and report it immediately. Also look for rales, shortness of breath, EKG changes, and distended neck veins. All of these signs may point to circulatory overload and you should report them immediately. Of course, you need to watch intravenous fluid rates carefully and continue to keep accurate intake and output records which include accurate daily weights.

"Third spacing" is an interesting and important phenomenon you are sure to hear more about as time goes on. It's another area of nursing in which you need to understand the physiology of normal fluid dynamics and know how to recognize changes in fluid distribution.

Edema
WHAT TO DO ABOUT IT

5

BY CATHERINE CIAVERELLI MANZI, RN

WITH THE WIDESPREAD USE of various drugs and hormonal agents, you're probably seeing more patients with edema than ever before. In some of these patients, edema has grave implications; in others, it may be insignificant. You need to know how to recognize both kinds and what to do about them.

Undoubtedly, you are most familiar with pulmonary edema, the most dangerous kind. Eleanore Lattimer, a 50-year-old artist, had pulmonary edema in its characteristic form. She was brought to the E.D. because of extreme shortness of breath.

She had hypertension for 15 years and was taking hydrochlorothiazide (HydroDIURIL) 50 mg twice a day and methyldopa (Aldomet) 250 mg four times a day. Two weeks before her admission she ran out of these medications. A few days later, she noticed dyspnea on exertion (when walking one block or climbing one flight of stairs) and also had swelling of both legs. During the night, she awakened with shortness of breath several hours after retiring. On the night of admission, she had become very short of breath and coughed up white foam.

Physical examination revealed an anxious, diaphoretic

woman who was severely short of breath. Her blood pressure was 220/120; pulse, 100; and respiratory rate, 44. Her neck veins distended when she sat up. She had bilateral diffuse, moist rales, and wheezing throughout both lungs. The cardiac examination showed an S_3 and S_4 gallop, and there was 4+ pitting edema of both legs.

The doctor diagnosed congestive heart failure with pulmonary edema. He ordered nasal oxygen at 6 liters per minute and an intravenous line with dextrose. Furosemide (Lasix) 80 mg and digoxin 0.5 mg were given I.V. push; morphine sulfate, 8 mg, was given slowly through the I.V.; and aminophylline, 250 mg in 100 ml 5% dextrose in water, was started to run in over 30 minutes. Rotating tourniquets were applied, and a Foley catheter was inserted so that her urine output could be accurately measured. IPPB by mask was also started.

She was transferred to the ICU. Over the next 2 hours, she had a urinary output of 1500 ml, and was much improved. The next day, she was started on a diuretic to alleviate her leg edema and maintenance digoxin (Lanoxin) to control her heart failure.

Not all forms of edema are as serious as Mrs. Lattimer's, whose condition was due to heart failure. You know that certain drugs, notably oral contraceptives, can cause relatively benign fluid retention. But however mild the accumulation of fluid may seem, if either you or your patient notice swelling, it's clinical edema and you need to deal with it. And that doesn't always take diuretics or other intervention. Before you can try to alleviate edema, you must know what's causing it.

How edema happens

Edema reflects sodium retention, which can result from excessive reabsorption (heart failure, cirrhosis) or inadequate elimination because of failing renal function (nephrotic syndrome, acute glomerulonephritis, acute tubular necrosis, or chronic renal disease). But that's not all. In congestive failure, another contributing mechanism is increased hydrostatic pressure at the capillary membranes which causes fluid to accumulate in the tissues.

But the chain of internal events doesn't stop there. If fluid loss in the capillary bed is severe, the resulting hypovolemia decreases kidney perfusion which, in turn, stimulates renin

1 SLIGHT, +1 PITTING EDEMA   **2** +4 PITTING EDEMA   **3** BRAWNY EDEMA

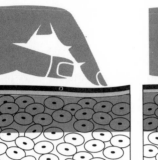 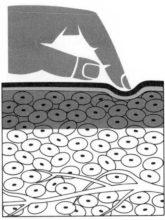 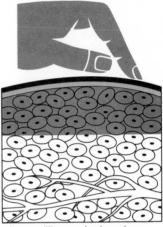

Evaluating edema

Pitting edema is evaluated on a four-point scale: from +1 (a barely detectable pit, as in Figure 1) to +4 (a deep and persistent pit, approximately 1 inch or 25.4 mm deep, as in Figure 2). An adult patient can accumulate up to 10 lb (4.5 kg) of fluid before you will be able to detect a pit. The skin pits against a bony surface, such as the subcutaneous aspect of the tibia, fibula, sacrum, or sternum.

Edema can become so severe that pitting is not possible; the tissue becomes so full that fluid can't be displaced. Subcutaneous tissue becomes fibrotic and as a result, the surface tissue feels rock hard. Over time this condition can develop into brawny edema (Figure 3). For example, a mastectomy patient whose axillary nodes have been removed may develop brawny edema in her affected arm. The patient's arm looks like a pig's skin, and becomes hard or gelatinous to the touch. Brawny edema can also indicate lymphatic obstruction.

Protect all edematous extremities from injury: A large quantity of edema makes the skin prone to sloughing and ulceration.

secretion. Renin triggers hypersecretion of aldosterone, which causes the patient to retain even more sodium and water. Thus, as more and more sodium is reabsorbed, less and less can be excreted. And massive edema can develop.

Recognize clinical edema

Watch for several reliable signs:

• *Pitting or brawny edema.* (See insert.)

• *Excessive weight gain* (a weight gain of 1 kg (2.2 lbs) equals 1 liter of fluid retention). To keep track of edema, weigh the patient daily, on the same scale, at the same time and in the same kind of clothes. Report any changes.

• *Elevated blood pressure* (which may have other causes).

• *Dyspnea* (which may or may not be present).

• *Neck vein distention* in upright position.

When you find any of the above signs, confirm clinical edema with laboratory tests. Look for:

- low hematocrit (the red blood cells are diluted in an excessive volume of extracellular fluid).
- low urine sodium (due to sodium retention).

Pulmonary edema an emergency

Pulmonary edema may grow out of the increased hydrostatic pressure associated with heart failure or the capillary injury in primary lung disease. Watch for early clues. The patient with pulmonary edema may not have visible edema anywhere else but is likely to have some telltale symptoms that warn you of his impending trouble:

Dyspnea on exertion is an early signal. So is *neck vein distention. Paroxysmal nocturnal dyspnea* comes later. The patient may tell you that he can only breathe easily in an upright position. Typically, he'll awake short of breath soon after retiring, insisting that he needs "fresh air." Ten or fifteen minutes after sitting up, he'll feel relieved. When such a patient needs to sleep on two to three pillows to overcome nocturnal dyspnea, he has developed *orthopnea,* a late symptom.

Keep in mind that the patient who's recently developed *nocturia* may have early congestive failure which could lead to pulmonary edema. His nocturia may be due to fluid shifts during the night while he's recumbent. The fluid that accumulates in the legs during the day is mobilized and excreted by the kidneys at night. Ultimately, when the patient's kidneys can no longer excrete enough of this excess fluid, he'll develop paroxysmal nocturnal dyspnea.

Unlike most other edematous patients, the patient with acute pulmonary edema must be treated immediately. His condition is a true emergency. In determining nursing care priorities, bear in mind these urgent needs:

- *The need to increase the concentration and transfer of oxygen across the alveolar membrane.* First make the patient comfortable in a sitting position. (Most patients with pulmonary edema voluntarily assume this position.) Then if there is no history of chronic obstructive pulmonary disease, administer high flow oxygen as ordered or oxygen by intermittent positive pressure. These measures help deliver needed oxygen across the alveoli and decrease venous return to the heart by increasing intrathoracic pressure.
- *The need to improve cardiac output and vascular circula-*

NEPHRON UNIT

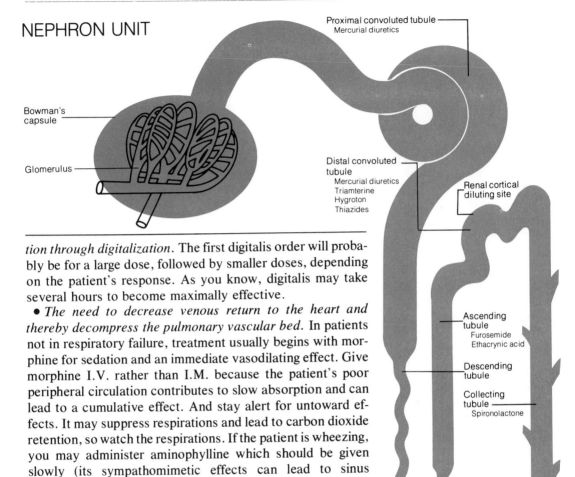

Proximal convoluted tubule
Mercurial diuretics

Bowman's
capsule

Glomerulus

Distal convoluted
tubule
Mercurial diuretics
Triamterine
Hygroton
Thiazides

Renal cortical
diluting site

Ascending
tubule
Furosemide
Ethacrynic acid

Descending
tubule

Collecting
tubule
Spironolactone

Loop of
Henle

tion through digitalization. The first digitalis order will probably be for a large dose, followed by smaller doses, depending on the patient's response. As you know, digitalis may take several hours to become maximally effective.

• *The need to decrease venous return to the heart and thereby decompress the pulmonary vascular bed.* In patients not in respiratory failure, treatment usually begins with morphine for sedation and an immediate vasodilating effect. Give morphine I.V. rather than I.M. because the patient's poor peripheral circulation contributes to slow absorption and can lead to a cumulative effect. And stay alert for untoward effects. It may suppress respirations and lead to carbon dioxide retention, so watch the respirations. If the patient is wheezing, you may administer aminophylline which should be given slowly (its sympathomimetic effects can lead to sinus tachycardia).

Some doctors feel the best way to relieve pulmonary congestion is to apply pneumatically driven, rotating tourniquets. Others prefer to do a phlebotomy.

• *The need to eliminate retained sodium and water.* One of the potent, rapidly acting diuretics (probably furosemide [Lasix]) will be ordered. It's usually administered I.V. to diurese the patient as quickly as possible. Diuresis should begin within 10 to 15 minutes. If diuresis hasn't yet occurred at the end of 2 hours, a larger dose of the diuretic may be needed. (But be careful: A patient's failure to respond may reflect renal disease or severely decreased cardiac output and inadequate renal blood flow.)

Where diuretics work
The drawing above shows where certain diuretics work within the nephron unit. Medical studies have found that the mercurials, furosemide, ethacrynic acid and the thiazides work at other sites as well.

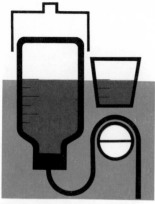

Nursing care of edematous extremities
- Keep skin clean and dry
- Protect from injury
  — while bathing or handling for any reason, do so gently and carefully
  — remove room equipment that could easily bump the edematous part (foot stools and the like)
  — avoid constrictive clothing (garters, elastic stockings)
- Keep edematous part elevated
- Observe for and record
  — sores and blisters
  — increasing size
  — absence of pulses
  — numbness
  — tingling
  — coldness
  — cyanosis

Edema often benign

Perhaps the most common edema is hormonal. It occurs during the menstrual life of many apparently healthy women who aren't pregnant. The ovarian steroids, particularly the estrogens, can encourage sodium retention and consequently cause generalized edema. When estrogen and progesterone secretion increase, as happens before a woman's menses, sodium and water are excessively retained, causing premenstrual edema. Women in their thirties and forties are particularly vulnerable to this cyclic edema, which is usually accompanied by headaches, irritability, and puffy feet. A moderately low sodium diet and a 1- or 2-day course of a thiazide before each menstrual period can help such women.

As you know, edema is a troublesome problem for women who use oral contraceptives because these synthetic steroids promote sodium and fluid retention. The higher the estrogen content of the medication, the more likely the patient is to develop edema. The same problem also plagues women in menopause who take synthetic or natural conjugated estrogen. There's not too much to be done about this kind of edema, other than reducing dosage or changing or discontinuing medication. But you need to be aware of it because it comes up so often.

Edema after stroke

Patients recuperating from stroke risk developing edema, generally on the paralyzed side. Edema occurs in such patients primarily because they're unable to perform the muscular activity required to pump blood through the venous system and its valves. With muscular activity gone, hydrostatic pressure rises at the venous end of the capillary, and lymph fluid accumulates. If the condition persists long enough, the patients will develop brawny edema.

So watch carefully for developing edema in stroke patients. Do whatever you can to improve peripheral circulation. For example, turn the bedridden patient frequently; do range-of-motion exercises to the affected side; and watch for sacral edema. Teach the patient and his family how to do special exercises to prevent brawny edema. Explain why they are important, and encourage and assist the patient to use a chair or wheelchair as much as possible.

A similar edema develops in post-mastectomy patients.

They, too, need to do special exercises. Explain why these exercises are so important. Watch the patient as she learns them to be sure she is doing them correctly.

Edema in pregnancy

A certain amount of edema is considered physiological during pregnancy. Increased circulating blood volume and increased tissue fluid account for it. So does a natural reduction in albumin (which lowers plasma colloid osmotic pressure). Furthermore, so do increases in estrogen, progesterone, and cortisone. A moderately low sodium diet can help pregnant women avoid undue edema. In the toxemia-prone patient, a low sodium diet helps lessen the severity of the toxemia and sometimes eliminates subsequent eclampsia.

If sodium restriction alone does not prevent edema in pregnant women, some obstetricians favor adding a thiazide diuretic. Treatment usually lasts 2 to 3 days, with intermittent lapses of a day or two to avoid potassium depletion. Such patients are advised to take the diuretic in the morning, so that their nighttime rest will not be disturbed by the need to void.

Side effects and hidden sources

Expect edema with certain drugs. Cortisone (Cortone), hydrocortisone (Cortef), prednisone (Deltasone), and prednisolone (Delta-Cortef) are more likely to cause edema than the fluorinated congeners (triamcinolone [Aristocort], dexamethasone [Decadron], and betamethasone [Celestone] have little or no mineralocorticoid activity). Several non-hormonal drugs may also cause edema. Two anti-inflammatory agents — phenylbutazone (Butazolidin) and its analogue, oxyphenbutazone (Tandearil) — do so, as does the antihypertensive agent, guanethidine sulfate (Ismelin).

A skimpy or inadequate diet leads to hypoproteinemia and therefore edema. Poor and elderly people are the chief victims of hypoproteinemia, but so are some patients with liver, kidney, or gastrointestinal problems. For example, alcoholics may have hypoproteinemia secondary to cirrhosis.

How about the patient whose edema seems unresponsive to diet and diuretics? He may, in fact, be getting extra sodium inadvertently. You can help by reviewing with him the foods that are high in sodium, including the not-so-obvious ones. His concept of a restricted sodium diet may be way off base. He

What's cooking?
Here are some helpful food suggestions for the patient with fluid problems controlled by a diuretic. These foods are high in potassium but low in sodium.
FRUITS AND THEIR JUICES
Apples
Apricots
Bananas
Dates
Grapefruit
Nectarines
Oranges
Prunes
Raisins
Watermelon
VEGETABLES (fresh or frozen)
Asparagus
Beans
Brussels sprouts
Cabbage
Cauliflower
Corn
Lima beans
Peas
Peppers
Potatoes
Radishes
Squash

may realize the saltiness of foods such as anchovies, soy sauce and pretzels, but not that of carbonated beverages, commercial breads, canned soups and delicatessen meats. Help the patient plan some simple meals. If he's hospitalized, watch his meal tray for salt; and make sure he gets the right tray and the right diet.

Another hidden source of sodium is the drinking water of certain areas of the country. Coastal water supplies sometimes contain excess sodium; so do those in hard-water areas where softeners are used. Water softeners can *add* more than 150 mg/L to the sodium content.

When are diuretics needed? First of all, most patients with edema don't need diuretics at all. Edema itself is usually harmless, and most edematous patients shouldn't be hurriedly treated until the cause of their edema is determined. Sometimes, edema represents the body's effort to correct a physiologic imbalance. If so, too vigorous a diuresis or salt and water deprivation will interfere with the body's ability to maintain intravascular volume, and will do more harm than good.

Of course, in edema of renal or cardiac origin, the patient's sodium intake must be strictly controlled and diuretics are usually needed. How low can you reduce your patient's dietary sodium? A daily sodium intake of 1,000 mg is about as low as most ambulatory patients can follow successfully. Explain to chronic renal and cardiac patients how diet and diuretics control the amount of sodium in their bodies. Teach them to use a sphygmomanometer, so they can check and record their blood pressure daily. If they weigh themselves daily (Warn them to weigh themselves at the same time, in the same kind of clothes, and on the same scale.), they'll soon see that any sudden changes in these are directly related to their sodium intake. Some doctors feel that the patient who keeps his daily record of weight and blood pressure can learn to adjust the amount of diuretic he needs according to what the scale and mercury column tell him.

When a patient with chronic kidney failure reaches the stage where he can't readily excrete sodium and water, diuretics are no longer useful. Then the only line of defense is to eliminate sodium intake totally.

Edema needn't cause much concern unless it's a sign of heart failure, preeclampsia or pulmonary edema. Then your prompt attention can avert serious problems.

Dehydration
WHEN TO LOOK FOR IT

BY LAVENIA COLEMAN, RN

IF YOU OFTEN CARE for the elderly or for febrile infants and children, you know how common and troublesome dehydration can be. But dehydration is not confined to these two groups so notoriously vulnerable to it. It occurs in patients of all ages.

You've probably seen many patients like Mrs. Melendez. Mrs. Melendez, a 47-year-old salesclerk, was admitted through the emergency department because of nausea, vomiting, and diarrhea of 2 days' duration. She'd been in her usual good health until 2 days before admission. She had no history of similar episodes, ulcer disease, or alcohol use. She denied weight loss or a change in bowel habits. There was nothing to suggest toxic ingestion or food poisoning.

At physical examination, she was slightly lethargic and febrile (101° F. [38.3° C.] rectally); her skin was dry; her chest was clear; and her abdomen was slightly distended but nontender. Rectal examination revealed the presence of stool and mucus which were grossly hematest positive. The doctor's diagnosis was dehydration secondary to severe gastroenteritis or pyloric obstruction. He inserted a nasogastric tube to low Gomco suction. Nasogastric aspiration was clear, with

Water signs?

To help you assess your patient's condition, here's a list of signs and symptoms of fluid loss and excess:

WATER LOSS

Symptoms
  Dizziness, weakness
  Thirst, inability to swallow dry food
  Difficulty speaking

Signs
  Dry skin and mucous membranes
  Swollen, dry, and fissured tongue
  Postural hypotension, fever
  Weight loss
  Increased serum hematocrit, sodium, osmolality
  Oliguria, anuria
  Urine sodium less than 10 mEq/L

WATER EXCESS

Symptoms
  Confusion, poor coordination
  Nausea
  Muscle cramps, weakness
  Headache

Signs
  Weight gain
  Intake greater than output
  Moist skin
  Edema (peripheral, systemic, pulmonary)
  Convulsions, coma
  Hypertension
  Elevated CVP
  Gallop (S3) heart sounds
  Bounding pulse
  Low serum sodium, hemoglobin, osmolality
  Ascites

hematest positive. Her X-ray (flat plate of the abdomen) was compatible with pyloric obstruction.

We took vital signs every 4 hours on the day of admission and, afterwards, after every shift. The doctor ordered bedrest and nothing by mouth. We started intake and output records. She received intravenous infusions: 3000 ml 5% dextrose in ½ normal saline with 20 mEq KCl/L over the first 24 hours.

On the third day, all of her symptoms subsided. Her nasogastric tube was removed and intravenous treatment was discontinued.

The next day, her lab findings were within normal limits and she was discharged. As is common with simple dehydration after prolonged vomiting, recovery followed replacement of lost fluid.

What causes dehydration?

Usually dehydration stems from inadequate intake of water due to inability to swallow, coma, or the unavailability of water. Even when no water is being taken in, certain obligatory losses continue relentlessly in about these daily amounts: respiration (600 ml), perspiration (400 ml), urine (500 ml). These losses are almost pure water, so the concentration of the extracellular fluid rises. (Indeed, with loss of any body fluid other than blood, more water is usually lost than electrolytes.)

You can cope with or even prevent dehydration if you know when to expect it and how to recognize it. Remember the special situations that lead to fluid loss: extreme debilitation and illness; mechanical devices and intubation; drainage from wounds and suctioning; burns and massive injuries; and coma, inability to swallow, and unavailability of water. Similarly, certain symptoms predispose to extreme fluid loss: fever, fluid shifts, vomiting, hemorrhage, and hyperventilation.

When you do suspect dehydration, watch for telltale changes in body temperature, vital signs, and skin tone. Because fever increases loss of body fluids, you need to record temperature elevations and report them promptly. The patient with prolonged fever needs increased intake of water and other nutrients. Low blood pressure readings are another clue to dehydration. As you assess the patient's condition, pay special attention to the appearance of his skin and the mucous membranes of his mouth. If you pull his skin up, does it resume normal position quickly when you let go? If not, he may be dehydrated. (But this isn't always a reliable sign in people who are old or very thin.)

When a patient like Mrs. Melendez is admitted to your floor, ask yourself the following questions and consider the answers in your care plan.

• *Has the patient been eating and drinking normally?* If not, how long has intake been deficient? The real test of nursing skill lies not in just ordering and serving the right diet and fluids but in getting the patient to eat and drink them. When encouraging fluids, remember that some fruit juices, tea, coffee, carbonated drinks, and water are better tolerated than sweet concentrated liquids (which often cause abdominal distention and loss of appetite).

• *Is the patient's diet restricted?* If so, how might it affect his fluid balance? Illness or imposed dietary restrictions may greatly decrease the patient's desire to eat. When at all possible, allow him choices within his diet, to increase his acceptance of it. (Many patients find dietary restrictions difficult and unless you try to make these restrictions more tolerable, they may stop eating altogether or cheat on the diet.) If you work in a hospital where the dietary department serves the meal trays, it's easy to forget that many patients need considerable help at mealtime. Personnel who deliver meals sometimes leave meal trays where patients can't reach them; and, they are likely to pick up and return trays to the kitchen without noticing or reporting that the food was untouched. So, at mealtime, check to see that patients who need help are getting it. Position them comfortably at mealtime; help them avoid unnecessary interruptions; make sure that food arrives warm (and is the correct diet); and provide whatever help they need in preparing food for eating. After meals, check the patients' trays to be sure they actually did eat.

• *Is the patient thirsty?* If he's a bit dehydrated, he'll be asking for water. But don't rely on thirst as the only indicator of need. The elderly patient doesn't always recognize thirst, and if he does, may be too weak to reach his water supply. Besides, he tends to develop personality changes and mental confusion along with fluid imbalances.

• *Has the patient been receiving any medication or treatment?* For example, steroids are likely to produce fluid volume excess (by their tendency to encourage retention of sodium and water and to excrete potassium). Diuretics, even

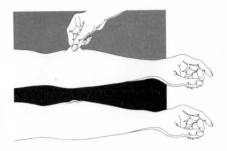

The pinch test
If you pinch the skin on a patient's forearm or sternum, under normal circumstances the skin will resume its shape quickly, within a few seconds. If the skin remains wrinkled for 20 to 30 seconds, however, the patient has poor skin turgor. Reduced or poor skin turgor may indicate dehydration, rapid weight reduction, or senile cutaneous atrophy. Report your findings to the doctor.

when taken correctly, may lead to electrolyte depletion.

• *If the patient has an abnormal fluid loss, what is its cause?*
Extracellular fluid volume deficit may follow severe vomiting or prolonged gastric suction which waste both water and electrolytes. Large open wounds and ascites can lead to similar fluid volume deficit.

Keep accurate intake and output records
Whenever you suspect an imbalance between intake and output or an electrolyte imbalance, you're responsible for charting intake and output on your own. Also alert the doctor to the potential fluid balance problem. Enlist the aid of the patient, if you can, and his family in helping keep the intake-output record accurate. When possible, measure all fluids directly. Estimate volumes only for fluids that cannot be measured directly; then record your estimates and, always, this information: fluid lost as perspiration; bed linen and clothing changes; uncaught or spilled vomitus; incontinent urine; fluid lost as liquid feces; and wound exudate (see also Chapter 3).

Sometimes you may be asked to assess the patient's state of hydration by measuring his urine's specific gravity. If so, you should learn how to carry out this procedure. However, the simplest way to keep track of the patient's fluid status is with accurate daily weights.

In certain situations such as oral surgery, swallowing problems, unconsciousness, and weakness caused by chronic debilitating conditions, oral intake may be impossible even though gastrointestinal function is adequate. Watch such patients carefully for inadequate intake and report it immediately. Do not wait for gross dehydration and malnutrition to develop before suggesting another route for nutrient intake. Obviously, such patients often need nasogastric feedings, total parenteral nutrition or intravenous therapy (see Chapters 22 and 23).

Acid-Base Imbalance
HOW TO RECOGNIZE IT

7

BY CARLA LEE, RN, BSN, MA

JUDY LONDERGAN, A 32-YEAR-OLD dress designer, was brought to the hospital one morning by her husband. She had cramping explosive diarrhea of 2 days' duration, and she complained of headache, nausea, drowsiness, and lethargy. Her eyes and cheeks looked sunken, suggesting a fluid deficit. She was hyperventilating, and her breath had a fruity odor.

Mrs. Londergan had been on a self-prescribed, high-fat, low-carbohydrate reducing diet for 3 weeks. She customarily took acetazolamide (Diamox) for 10 days before each menstrual period for premenstrual tension and edema. She had taken 250 mg a day of this diuretic for the past 9 days. About 48 hours before hospitalization, she had begun having diarrhea and occasional vomiting which she attributed to an "intestinal bug." She had no history of diabetes or renal disease.

What did Mrs. Londergan's laboratory results show? Despite her fruity breath, her fasting blood sugar was low at 60 mg per 100 ml. Her hematocrit was high, 54 ml/100 ml, confirming fluid deficit. And her other findings (see p. 68) pointed to metabolic acidosis. Mrs. Londergan had undergone a triple-barreled attack on her bicarbonate stores.

First, the 3-week reducing diet, in which she permitted no

more than 20 grams of carbohydrate daily, had produced the desired weight loss, but had induced ketosis. Excess ketones, coming from oxidation of fatty acids as a primary energy source, depress the plasma bicarbonate. Second, the acetazolamide designed to excrete bicarbonate through the urine, took sodium, water, and potassium with it. But because it is a carbonic anhydrase inhibitor, it prevented the easy formation of new bicarbonate stores. And finally, the heavy sacrifice of bowel fluids (a rich source of bicarbonate) tipped the scales toward full-blown acidosis.

When you see a patient like Mrs. Londergan, do you know how to determine if her distressed breathing (Kussmaul) is due to diabetic ketoacidosis, some other acid-base disturbance, or a combination of both? Mixed disturbances, in which two or more of the primary alterations coexist (for example, respiratory acidosis and metabolic alkalosis) are even more complex. With these disturbances, you may have to refer to a nomogram to separate the simple acid-base disturbance from a mixed one. However, arterial blood pH, CO_2 combining power of the venous blood, and recognition of the underlying disease will help you to identify it correctly.

Can you anticipate the treatment the doctor will order, so that you can be ready to give it promptly? When giving such treatment do you know what problems to expect and how to avoid them? If not, you may benefit from the following review of acid-base balance and its clinical implications.

What causes metabolic acidosis?
Metabolic acidosis results from either a primary base deficit (loss of bicarbonate) or an accumulation of fixed acids (acids created in metabolism). Many forms of metabolic acidosis are characterized by an abnormal anion gap (see p. 69). In Mrs. Londergan's case, both these factors contributed. Her low carbohydrate intake caused an increase in fat metabolism. The by-product of fat metabolism is excess acid production.

Metabolic acidosis usually results from:

• *Excessive burning of fats*. The major accumulants are ketoacids caused by excessive catabolism of fats in the absence of usable carbohydrate (diabetic ketoacidosis, for example). A diabetic has little or no insulin available to move glucose into the cells to be converted to energy. This means *high blood sugar* and glycosuria. But with *low intracellular sugar,* the cells, lacking sugar, burn fat. But fats are consumed far more rapidly than enzymes can handle the end products; ketone bodies are produced in excess.

The kidneys try to excrete the excess as acetone; the lungs try through Kussmaul respiration — fast, labored, deep breathing — to inactivate some of the excess H^+. They do this by expelling carbon dioxide — as well as enough acetone to lend its odor to the breath. But eventually the excess overtakes the compensation, and diabetic ketoacidosis results.

Malnutrition also produces ketones in the blood when the body has burned all the glycogen stores in the liver. So do low carbohydrate diets.

• *Abnormal carbohydrate metabolism.* Here, lactic acid accumulates from metabolism of carbohydrates in the absence of oxygen. Hypoxia, often caused by shock, permits glucose to be incompletely metabolized into lactic acid rather than carbon dioxide and water. Both buffers and lungs will try to compensate for that. Both the oxygen insufficiency at the cellular level and the attempted respiratory compensation will produce the fast breathing typical of shock. Of course, shock doesn't necessarily produce lactic acidosis. If you watch for it, you can usually prevent lactic acidosis.

• *Inadequate excretion of fixed-acid products of metabolism.* Renal insufficiency is the usual cause of acid retention. These acids appear in the blood serum as urea nitrogen, creatinine, and uric acid. Like the blood, the urine pH becomes more acidic with excretion of excessive amounts of both normal and abnormal acids. So, always watch patients with advancing renal disease carefully for acidosis.

• *And some other causes.* Losses of certain electrolytes, such as bicarbonate, also cause acidosis. Much of the loss in diarrhea comes from the pancreas, which habitually pours large amounts of alkali (also carrying digestive enzymes) into the small intestines to neutralize the escaping stomach acids. Rapid peristalsis intensifies this loss. So does pancreatic fistula, ileostomy, and duodenal fistula.

The terminal stage of Addison's disease leads to acidosis from loss of sodium chloride. As you know, when sodium is lost, potassium is usually retained. If serum potassium levels rise abnormally, the cells start to absorb it, releasing hydrogen into the blood in exchange and producing acidemia. Excessive intake of aspirin — acetylsalicylic acid — can also cause

The anion gap

The anion gap, or delta, represents the presence of lactate, pyruvate, acetate, and other anions that aren't measured in the typical electrolyte battery. You can estimate the anion gap using the concentrations of sodium, chloride, and bicarbonate, although what actually determines the anion gap is the concentration of unmeasured anions and unmeasured cations.

The calculation of the anion gap is based on the concept that total serum cations equal total serum anions. In this equation total serum cations consist of sodium and unmeasured cations (UC); total serum anions consist of chloride, bicarbonate, and unmeasured anions. This equation can be expressed chemically:

$Na + UC = (Cl + HCO_3) + UA$ or

$Na - (Cl + HCO_3) = UA - UC$

Substituting normal values,

$Na (145) - [Cl (109) + HCO_3 (26)]$

$=$ the anion gap

The normal anion gap is 10 to 12 mEq/L. It should always be less than 14. If it isn't, the patient suffers metabolic acidosis. In some cases, acidosis can coexist with a normal anion gap, as in cases of diarrhea, renal tubular acidosis or in patients receiving acidifying agents or carbonic anhydrase inhibitors.

Potassium in acidosis

Serum potassium value, in acidosis, does not offer much of a clue to total body potassium. In chemical buffering, hydrogen moves into the cells in exchange for potassium. The potassium thus released causes a rise in serum potassium which needs careful watching and, above 6.0 mEq/L, treatment. So in the first few hours watch for general weakness, malaise, muscle irritability, flaccid paralysis, as well as nausea, intestinal colic, and diarrhea. Correcting the acidosis will send needed potassium back into the cells. But, by then, much stored potassium will have been lost through the urine. With reentry into the cells, potassium serum levels will start to fall. So as treatment proceeds, potassium levels may fall low enough to need supplementing, although this should be done only if there is adequate urine flow. If untreated, potassium levels may drop sharply enough to be dangerous. Watch for diminished reflexes, weak pulse, and falling blood pressure. This may go with shallow breathing, shortness of breath and, again, vomiting.

metabolic acidosis, in the late stages of intoxication. So, as we have seen with Mrs. Londergan, can overzealous use of Diamox and improper diet.

Clues for assessment

Three major systems of the body offer clues to acidosis: the neurological, the gastrointestinal, and the respiratory. Early in acidosis, the patient may complain of headache and lethargy. As the acid level continues to rise, lethargy deepens into drowsiness. Untreated, this will lead to stupor, semi-consciousness, coma, and death. Other signs to look for include: fruity breath, anorexia, and nausea progressing to vomiting, diarrhea, and hyperventilation. This last comes from stimulation of the hypothalamus by the excess acid.

What lab values to expect? Low blood pH; the total CO_2 of the serum — measuring circulating bicarbonate — may be below 22 mEq/L. If the lungs are compensating for the acidosis by successfully venting enough carbon dioxide, its blood measurement (PCO_2) will fall below the normal 34 mm Hg.

Correction of acidosis from *renal failure* requires peritoneal or hemodialysis and low-protein, high-calorie diets. For lactic acidosis, oxygen and large doses of sodium bicarbonate are given. For Addison's disease, steroid therapy is given, along with extra salt.

In Mrs. Londergan's case, treatment began with an intravenous infusion of lactated Ringer's solution with 5% dextrose. And 44.6 mEq of sodium bicarbonate was added piggyback. The nurse kept a 4-hour check on potassium levels. Although serum levels were high at first, correction of the acidosis later drove these stores back into the cells twice depleted of potassium, once from biological regulation, again from diuresis. Potassium was added to the I.V. for infusion at a very slow rate. Had her fasting blood sugar been higher, regular insulin probably would have been given as a rapid treatment for hyperkalemia.

Acidosis often preventable

To correct acidosis, teach your diabetic patients to routinely test their urine for sugar and acetone; and to correctly use diet, insulin, and oral hypoglycemics. And watch carefully for acidosis in diabetic patients receiving I.V.s that could upset their acid-base balance; and in those with shock, hyperthyroidism, liver disease, advanced circulatory failure, intestinal or biliary intubation, or fluid deficit, or those who have been given acidifying salts.

Unfortunately, too many patients come to the hospital only after critical depletion of the chemical buffer system makes them feel terrible. By that time, acidosis is already serious. Then, the quickest way to overcome dangerous acidosis may be to replenish the supply of chemical buffers by giving intravenous bicarbonate or its forerunner, lactate. The usual dose is 1 to 3 ampules of sodium bicarbonate solution (44.6 mEq per ampule).

Three causes of alkalosis

Metabolic alkalosis has three basic causes: the uncompensated loss of acids, the retention (or ingestion) of too much base, and radical changes in the body's potassium level.

Loss of acids can come from vomiting, drainage by nasogastric tube, gavage, and fistulae. Acids are lost through the kidneys by potent diuretics (furosemide [Lasix], and ethacrynic acid [Edecrin]). Steroids can also lead to alkalosis. They cause sodium and chloride to be retained; potassium and hydrogen to be excreted.

Retention of alkali usually results from improper medication. Taking bicarbonate of soda and other alkalizing agents for an "acid stomach" leads the list. I.V. fluids high in bicarbonate rank high on this list — which also includes giving too much sodium bicarbonate during an emergency; Ringer's lactate; and solutions containing acetate and citrate (excessive transfusion with citrated blood).

Hypokalemia accompanies alkalosis. When hydrogen ions are low, as they are in alkalemia, the cells — to help regulate the base level — release H^+ into the serum in exchange for potassium, creating a serum deficit of potassium.

Clues to assessment

In metabolic alkalosis, blood tests usually show a pH above 7.45. The total serum content of CO_2 (telling of circulating base bicarbonate levels) rises above 32 mEq/L. The PCO_2 will not change unless the lungs are helping to compensate for the alkalosis by retaining carbon dioxide; then it will rise. In one kind of metabolic alkalosis, hypochloremic alkalosis (see Chapter 12), gastric losses of chloride greatly exceed the loss of

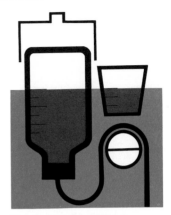

Nursing tips for acidosis
• *Check vital signs frequently.* Expect a rise in pulse rate as the body compensates. In diabetic acidotic patients, blood pressure drops because of hypovolemia. Stay alert for arrhythmias from hyperkalemia.
• *Chart intake and output precisely.* The doctor must know how the kidneys are functioning to plan effective treatment.
• *Begin safety and seizure precautions* as soon as the patient shows any decompensating neurologic changes such as twitching, stupor, or coma. Because vomiting is common in acidosis, position him on his side so he won't aspirate the vomitus. In many hospitals, a nasogastric tube connected to a low Gomco is customary, to prevent aspiration and to draw off excess acids and gases that build up in this acute state. If they were to accumulate from hypotonicity, gastric dilatation could complicate things.
• *Give good oral care.* But when you do, try not to stimulate the gag reflex. An alkaline mouthwash such as baking soda in water will help neutralize mouth acids, and lemon and glycerine swabs will help lubricate lips that are dried out by hyperpnea.
• *Teach the patient and his family* what they need to know about acidosis.

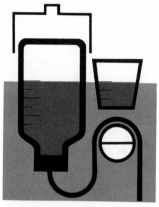

Nursing tips for alkalosis
Here are pointers for looking after the patient in metabolic alkalosis:
• *Take vital signs.* Hypotension and tachycardia suggest hypokalemia. Watch the respiratory rate, too. It will be decreased in compensation.
• *Tabulate intake and output.* This is needed for planning the replacement of lost electrolytes and fluids.
• As in acidosis, *take safety and seizure precautions* because these patients may be confused. Watch for early signs of neural irritability such as Trousseau's sign, which you can observe while you are taking the blood pressure. When the hand shows carpopedal spasm as you tighten the blood pressure cuff, this means tetany from calcium ion deficit in the alkalotic blood.
• *Check for muscle weakness,* too, from hypokalemia. You can see weakness of motion while bathing the patient, or during dangling and ambulation. If you notice any slowing down or decreased energy of movement, report it to the doctor.

sodium because of a corresponding increase in potassium loss. If cellular buffering has occurred, the serum potassium level will fall below 3.0 mEq/L.

As in acidosis the major systems to observe are neurological, gastrointestinal, and respiratory. An alkalotic patient will act fidgety, twitching and shaking, often picking at the sheets. He may be confused or irritable. He may develop tetany, flapping tremor (asterixis), convulsions, or coma.

The alkalotic patient is also susceptible to atrial tachycardias. His EKG usually shows a low T wave that, in later stages, merges with the P wave. He often develops nausea, vomiting, and diarrhea. The vomiting itself aggravates the alkalosis by sacrificing chlorides. His lungs try to compensate for metabolic alkalosis just as they do for acidosis; but in alkalosis, respirations are shallow and slow — an attempt to build up carbonic acid stores to neutralize the excess base.

Because alkalosis is chiefly induced by medication or postoperative losses, alert nursing care can often fend it off. First, warn your patients against dosing themselves needlessly with antacids. However, once a patient is alkalotic, the best treatment is to correct the underlying cause. Emergency therapy means giving acidifying I.V.s such as ammonium chloride or arginine hydrochloride which contains releasable hydrogen ions. Although ammonium chloride can correct the alkalosis, it must be given with extreme caution, for it can be hazardous. It can cause hyperchloremic metabolic acidosis, especially in patients with renal or liver impairment.

When the underlying problem is gastric loss, giving potassium chloride and normal saline will correct it: Replacement of excessive potassium losses frees hydrogen ions from the cells. Raising serum chloride levels promotes excretion of bicarbonate. Diuretic-induced alkalosis, often asymptomatic, can usually be treated merely by discontinuing the diuretic and replacing potassium and chloride. When resupplying potassium and chloride, replacement is best gauged by the amounts lost in secretions (such as 5 to 10 mEq of potassium per liter of gastric fluid). In any case, potassium should always be well diluted and given no faster than 20 mEq/hr, or no stronger than 80 mEq per liter of I.V. fluid unless hypokalemia is very severe (serum potassium less than 2.0 mEq/L). Monitor the EKG for potassium-induced arrhythmias, and check urine output frequently.

Respiratory acidosis

This kind of acidosis follows some failure of ventilation. It may come from: oversedation; head trauma that damages the medullary respiratory centers; paralysis of the muscles of respiration (poliomyelitis); upper-airway obstruction; acute involvement of the lung or bronchial tissues (infection, pulmonary edema, pneumonia, or atelectasis); chronic conditions (bronchiectasis, emphysema, or asthma); or, prolonged overbreathing of carbon dioxide.

Respiratory acidosis develops simply because too much carbon dioxide is retained. In either respiratory acidosis or respiratory alkalosis, the lungs fail in their regulatory function, and the remaining systems try to compensate.

There are two kinds of respiratory acidosis, acute and chronic. Patients with *acute respiratory acidosis* do not benefit greatly from the compensatory mechanisms. For one thing, the kidneys require several hours to several days to stabilize the acidosis. For another, the blood buffers and cellular chemical buffer require normal blood circulation and efficient tissue perfusion. In acute respiratory failure, an emergency airway has to be established before treatment can be started.

Chronic respiratory acidosis does respond well to compensation by the kidneys. It usually results from chronic obstructive lung disease. In such cases, the kidneys have enough time to compensate by abnormally retaining bicarbonate and can keep pH close to normal on the acid side in spite of an increased carbon dioxide. But such a patient has no leeway left. He can become acutely acidotic just by catching cold.

Clues to assessment

Laboratory tests show a blood pH below the normal 7.35 and a PCO_2 above the normal 46 mmHg. If the kidneys or other regulators are not compensating, bicarbonate (measured as serum CO_2 combining power) will remain normal. If they *are* compensating, it will go up, and so will potassium as it changes places with hydrogen — by coming out through the cell walls.

The patient in full-blown respiratory acidosis shows dulled sensorium, and restlessness and apprehension which can progress to somnolence, coma, or asterixis. During early phases, he will perspire and have a rapid pulse. If his condition becomes critical, he may become cyanotic. But don't wait to

Treatment critical

The first 24 to 48 hours are critical for the patient acutely ill with respiratory acidosis. Treatment must provide an airway, and maintain adequate ventilation and hydration. Endotracheal tube or tracheostomy may be needed for breathing. Intermittent positive pressure breathing (IPPB) may be ordered. The increased ventilation it provides may keep a somnolent, acidotic patient from succumbing to carbon dioxide narcosis.

Antibiotics may be ordered to eliminate any infection. But narcotics, hypnotics, and tranquilizers must be avoided because they further depress the respiratory center.

In chronic respiratory acidosis, the carbon dioxide stimulus ceases after a while to affect the respiratory centers, and oxygen deficit is the only remaining stimulus to breathe. *Never* risk removing this stimulus by giving more than 1 to 2 liters of oxygen per minute by cannula unless it is specifically ordered and its need shown by blood-gas determination. Then stand by. Otherwise, adhere strictly to low flow correlated with blood gas studies.

Pointers for further care:
Keep your patient under constant surveillance. Abrupt changes are too likely in the acute condition. Report signs of respiratory distress at once. Be ready to give cardiopulmonary resuscitation should the patient stop breathing.

Suctioning is important: It removes secretions that otherwise obstruct the airway. Encourage fluid intake; it can help thin the secretions. Give chest physiotherapy to loosen secretions, too. Postural drainage will help remove secretions by gravity.

Treatment supportive

Treatment of respiratory alkalosis is usually based on eliminating the underlying cause, which is frequently hysteria. It includes reassurance, sedation, and sometimes carbon dioxide inhalation. For the person whose respiratory alkalosis is neurogenic, breathing into a paper bag can help because he is rebreathing the carbon dioxide he has just exhaled along with partially deoxygenated air. This recycled carbon dioxide can eventually restore normal carbonic acid levels to the blood. Encouraging the patient to hold his breath can also help.

When caring for the patient who is hyperventilating, give the medication ordered and watch for signs of other disease that the respiratory alkalosis may be masking. This might include recognizing situations that could excite a patient to hysteria, and helping him cope with them before they arise. If prevention is no longer possible, give emotional support; often this alone relieves hyperventilation.

look for cyanosis in such patients, because it's a *late* sign.

The patient with respiratory acidosis from chronic disease will at first breathe faster in an attempt to correct the actual decrease in ventilation. But after a while, he will breathe more and more slowly with prolonged expiration. If acutely ill, his respiratory center may stop responding to the higher carbon dioxide levels and he will abruptly stop breathing.

Respiratory alkalosis

Respiratory alkalosis occurs because of excessive venting of carbon dioxide through hyperventilation. The causes of hyperventilation include lack of oxygen, pulmonary embolus, high altitude, high environmental temperature, fever, infections, encephalitis, drug toxicity (early stages of salicylate poisoning), reactions to sulfanilamide, quinine, phenol, or antihistamine, and hysteria. Even voluntary overbreathing can cause it.

Chemical and chemical-cellular buffering are the major forms of compensation. The hydrogen-potassium shift that occurs here is the same as in metabolic alkalosis, with hydrogen coming out of the cells into the blood stream in exchange for potassium — creating a serum potassium deficiency. If alkalosis continues, the kidneys compensate by cutting back tubular acid losses and bicarbonate reabsorption.

Clues to assessment

Lab tests that point to respiratory alkalosis include a rise in the blood pH above 7.45; a decrease in the PCO_2 below 34 mm Hg; and a normal bicarbonate reading if the alkalosis is not compensated, or low reading if it is. The potassium level will be lower than normal. The best sign of respiratory alkalosis is deep, rapid breathing — sometimes above 40 respirations a minute and much like the Kussmaul breathing of the diabetic in acidosis. But while Kussmaul breathing tries to compensate for acidosis, this breathing causes it.

The hysterical patient generally shows anxiety and fear. He may have numbness and tingling of the hands and face besides. If alkalosis is due to pneumonia, salicylate intoxication, brain trauma, or pain, the emotional state can also have much to do with whether or not respiratory alkalosis appears. Incidentally, overzealous use of mechanical ventilators can also induce respiratory alkalosis.

SKILLCHECK 2

1. Mr. Eric Winter, a 53-year-old house painter, was admitted to the hospital with small-bowel obstruction. He gave a history of colicky abdominal pain, some watery diarrhea, and generalized abdominal tenderness for the past 3 days. At admission, he was noticeably anxious, his skin was pale, cool and clammy, and he was breathing rapidly. His pulse was rapid, urine was scanty and concentrated, and his abdomen was distended. A CVP line, Foley catheter, and nasogastric tube were quickly inserted and rapid I.V. infusions with lactated Ringer's solution were started in preparation for the O.R. Was Mr. Winter hypervolemic, hypovolemic, or alkalotic? How would you plan his management before and after surgery?

2. Mrs. Sarah Owens, a 69-year-old woman is admitted with chronic renal failure. Although the doctor has ordered strict intake and output, Mrs. Owens is incontinent during the night. During the day, despite constant reminders, she frequently forgets to save her urine for the nurse to measure. Your intake and output record will necessarily be inaccurate. How can you assess Mrs. Owens' fluid status?

3. *True or false.* Liver disease predisposes to abnormal retention of sodium and water. Explain why.

4. Mrs. Margaret Peters, a 79-year-old retired bookkeeper, was admitted for treatment of viral pneumonia. After several days in the hospital, she seemed to get more and more confused. One evening, she scratched one of the nurses and began to yell and scream, keeping the other patients awake. Her doctor was called and arterial blood gases were drawn. Blood gases did not show hypoxemia. She was sedated with Valium 5 mg p.o. On morning rounds, her nurse was unable to arouse her. Mrs. Peters' BP was stable, but she was tachycardic (120) and tachypneic (40). Arterial blood gases were drawn again, and this time revealed acute respiratory acidosis (pH, 7.32; PCO_2, 60 mmHg; and HCO_3^-, 27 mEq/L. What caused the acidosis?

5. Gerald James is a 24-year-old student hospitalized with a gunshot wound of his abdomen after a hunting accident. Three days ago, he had surgery to repair a perforated ileum and torn small bowel. He has a Dennis tube in place, and his condition has been stable. But this morning, he is complaining of abdominal pain and "not feeling right." You notice that his abdomen looks distended even though his tube is functioning properly. You take his vital signs and find that his pulse has risen from 88 to 110 beats per minute; his BP has fallen from 130/80 to 100/60. What could be wrong?

6. Mrs. Betty Lynn, a 50-year-old woman with coronary artery disease and chronic congestive failure, complained of paroxysmal nocturnal dyspnea. She'd been taking digitalis and HydroDIURIL, and had been on a 1000 mg Na restriction for many years. Her heart failure had been under good control. But for the last 3 weeks, she'd begun to wake up extremely short of breath about 2 to 3 hours after retiring. If she got out of bed, and sat for about 30 minutes, the dyspnea disappeared, and she could return to bed. She also noticed leg and ankle edema, late in the afternoon. She denied increased sodium intake, and firmly said she'd taken all her medications as directed. She then mentioned having recently begun to go through menopause, and had been severely distressed by frequent hot flashes. Her family doctor had prescribed an estrogen to relieve these symptoms. Too, she tearfully said that her husband who had recently lost his job had begun to drink heavily.

What is causing Mrs. Lynn's sudden paroxysmal nocturnal dyspnea? What can be done about it?

7. Mrs. Cooper, a 50-year-old widow with bronchogenic carcinoma, was admitted to the hospital from a nursing home. She had been complaining of anorexia and nausea, so an I.V. of 5% dextrose in water had been started at the nursing home. On admission, she was extremely weak, confused, and had muscle twitching. She was hypotensive. *Stat* electrolytes determinations were ordered, and showed that Mrs. Cooper was hyponatremic with a serum sodium of 120 mEq/L. She was thought to have inappropriate ADH secretion, probably triggered by the lung cancer, stress, and the morphine she was receiving for pain every 4 to 6 hours. The I.V. infusions of 5% dextrose in water caused water overload and produced dilutional hyponatremia. Mrs. Cooper's fluids were restricted, and I.V. furosemide (Lasix) was to be given after an infusion of 500 ml of 3% NaCl was started. The I.V. was to run 12 hours. Another nurse just finishing her shift, merely hung another bottle of 500 ml of 3% NaCl. The next shift nurse making her early rounds checked Mrs. Cooper's I.V. She immediately discontinued the 3% NaCl and called the doctor. Why?

(Answers on page 198)

MONITORING ELECTROLYTES

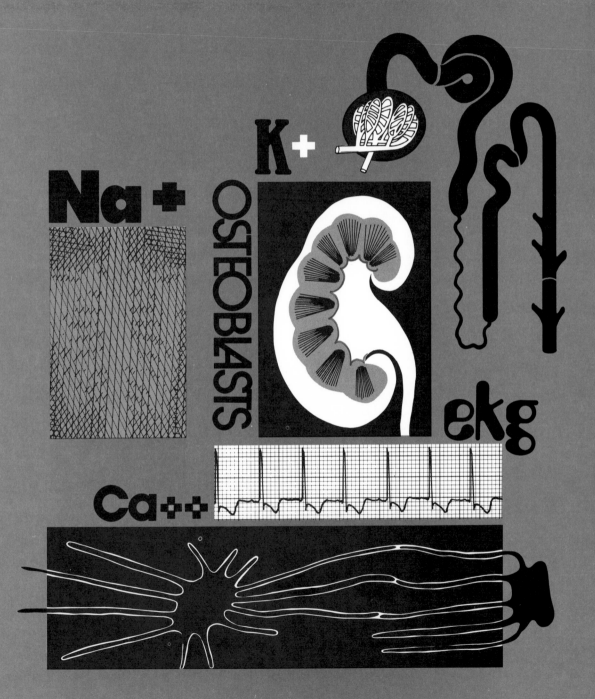

Potassium
THE CHIEF ELECTROLYTE

BY GRETCHEN REED, RN, BS, MA

IF YOU OFTEN SEE PATIENTS with cardiovascular problems, you know that diuretics are notorious wasters of potassium and that potassium depletion (hypokalemia) can exaggerate response to digitalis. The opposite condition, potassium excess (hyperkalemia), can induce symptoms even more catastrophic — first tachycardia, then bradycardia, then standstill.

To complicate matters, in many clinical situations, initial deficit can shift into excess; and excess into deficit. All of these things can develop slowly or abruptly. Clearly, in nursing, you need a working knowledge of potassium's clinical effects, to quickly recognize a potassium imbalance and deal with it correctly and promptly.

Why is potassium so important? Because it's the dominant cellular electrolyte and, thus, controls cellular osmotic pressure. Further, potassium activates several enzymatic reactions; helps regulate acid-base balance; influences kidney function and structure (nephropathy can follow prolonged potassium deficit), and maintains neuromuscular excitability.

As you know, potassium exists normally in the serum within a very narrow range — 3.5 to 5.0 mEq/L. Small deviations in either direction can have disastrous consequences, particu-

Potassium ebb and flow

In healthy kidneys (see opposite page), potassium undergoes a constant process of reabsorption into the serum, and secretion back into the renal tubules. The glomeruli filter serum potassium into the proximal tubule. Between there and the distal convoluted tubule, potassium is reabsorbed back into the serum. At the distal convoluted tubule potassium is secreted into the tubules. Then, at the collecting tubule, both processes — reabsorption and secretion — happen at the same time. The kidneys then excrete potassium in the urine, usually in association with a balancing reabsorption of sodium in the serum.

Because the kidneys excrete almost all of the daily intake of potassium, the body is especially vulnerable to hypokalemia.

larly for persons already ill. Even in those who are reasonably well, potassium imbalance can quickly become surprisingly severe. You have surely seen many patients like Mrs. Graham, a 56-year-old teacher who was brought to the emergency department after fainting in the street. Her history revealed increasing weakness and nausea during preceding weeks. She was 40 pounds overweight and hypertensive, and had been taking a thiazide diuretic for several months. But she had not been taking a potassium supplement and had not been careful about dietary potassium. Physical examination showed depressed patellar reflexes, rapid pulse, and soft, unusually flabby muscles. Plasma potassium was found to be only 3 mEq/L. An electrocardiogram showed the characteristic pattern of potassium depletion.

Fortunately, potassium levels usually stay within normal limits despite a great fluctuation in fluid and electrolyte intake. Like other electrolytes, potassium constantly shifts among blood, cells, gastrointestinal fluids, and urine. The same shifting goes on in sweat and salivary glands as well. What influences this movement of potassium? Adrenal steroid hormones, changes in pH, and changes in blood sugar levels do. So do changes in blood sodium levels: There seems to be a reciprocal relation between sodium and potassium; *a large intake of sodium increases the loss of potassium, and vice versa.*

Kidney wastes potassium

Under the influence of the body's adrenal steroids, particularly aldosterone, the kidneys conserve sodium by excreting potassium even when both are in short supply. This wasting takes place in the distal renal tubules where sodium and potassium are essentially on opposite sides of the renal tubular epithelium. There, sodium ions pass from the tubular fluid into the cells while potassium ions (and hydrogen ions) pass from the cells into the tubular fluid. Potassium gets excreted as sodium gets reabsorbed. Under normal conditions, approximately 80% of filtered potassium is reabsorbed. These ions exchange on a one-to-one basis. In actual depletion, a little extra potassium may be reabsorbed on its way out, from the collecting ducts of the kidney.

Because the kidneys preferentially conserve sodium, especially under the influence of aldosterone, you are likely to see

NEPHRON UNIT

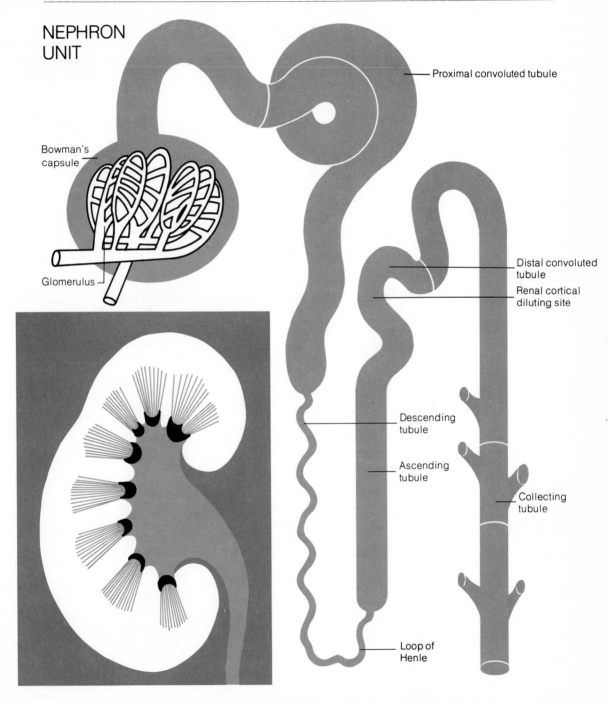

Proximal convoluted tubule

Bowman's capsule

Glomerulus

Distal convoluted tubule

Renal cortical diluting site

Descending tubule

Ascending tubule

Collecting tubule

Loop of Henle

Some Potassium Supplements

PRODUCT	AMOUNT OF POTASSIUM SUPPLIED (potassium chloride unless specified)	NURSING TIPS
Liquids Kay Ciel ◇ KCl-Rougier◇◇ K-10◇ Kaochlor 10% Kaochlor S-F Kay Ciel KLOR-10% Kloride Klorvess 10% Pan-kloride Pfiklor Rum-K Kaon-Cl 20% KLOR-CON Kaon Potassium-Rougier◇◇ Twin-K Duo-K Kolyum Potassium triplex	6.6 mEq/5 ml 10 mEq/15 ml 10% (20 mEq/15 ml) 10% (20 mEq/15 ml) 10% (20 mEq/15 ml) 10% (20 mEq/15 ml) 10% (20 mEq/15 ml) 10% (20 mEq/15 ml) 10% (20 mEq/15 ml) 10% (20 mEq/15 ml) 10% (20 mEq/15 ml) 15% (30 mEq/15 ml) 20% (40 mEq/ml) 20% (40 mEq/ml) 20 mEq/15 ml as gluconate 20 mEq/15 ml as gluconate 20 mEq gluconate and citrate 20 mEq potassium and 3.3 mEq chloride per 15 ml 20 mEq potassium and 3.3 mEq chloride per 15 ml 45 mEq/15 ml as acetate, bicarbonate, and citrate	• Due to many forms and varying amounts of potassium, give these supplements with extreme caution. Never switch potassium products without a doctor's order. If your patient tolerates one product better than another, tell the doctor so he can change the brand and dosage. • Give potassium in 2 to 4 doses per day over several days to avoid severe hyperkalemia. Give it with or after meals with a full glass of water or fruit juice to minimize GI irritation. Follow the manufacturer's recommendations for dilution. • Tell patients to sip liquid potassium products slowly to minimize GI irritation. Give to patients on fluid restriction at mealtime. Don't give to patients receiving potassium-sparing diuretics (spironolactone and triamterene).
Powders K-Lor Kato Kay Ciel K-Lor Pfiklor K-Lyte/Cl◇ Kolyum	15 mEq/packet 20 mEq/packet 20 mEq/packet 20 mEq/packet 20 mEq/packet 25 mEq/packet 20 mEq potassium and 3.34 mEq chloride per 5 g packet (gluconate and chloride)	• Make sure powders are *completely* dissolved. • A helpful tip: If patient's diet allows, mix total daily dose of potassium powder in boiling water and then add one packet of gelatin dessert, adding usual amount of cold water to the gelatin. Once the mixture sets, it can be divided into four servings or "doses."

Guide to drug charts
◇ available in Canada
◇◇ available in Canada only

	Some Potassium Supplements	
PRODUCT	AMOUNT OF POTASSIUM SUPPLIED (potassium chloride unless specified)	NURSING TIPS
Effervescent Tablets Kaochlor-Eff	20 mEq potassium and chloride (from potassium chloride, citrate, and bicarbonate and betaine HCl))	• Tell the patient to drink the solution after effervescence has subsided to minimize ingestion of HCO_3^-. Make sure the patient drinks all of the solution.
KEFF	20 mEq potassium and chloride (from potassium chloride, carbonate, and bicarbonate, and betaine HCl)	
Klorvess Pfiklor-F	20 mEq potassium and chloride (from potassium chloride and bicarbonate and l-lysine monohydrochloride)	
K-Lyte Potassium-Sandoz◇◇	25 mEq as bicarbonate and citrate 12 mEq potassium and 8 mEq of chloride (from chloride and bicarbonate)	
Tablets Potassium chloride	Enteric coated 300 mg (4 mEq); 650 mg (8.7 mEq); 1 g (13.4 mEq)	• Not recommended due to problems with GI bleeding and small bowel ulcerations.
Slow-K◇	Sugar-coated: 600 mg (8 mEq) in wax matrix	• Potassium chloride tablets in wax matrix have been known to lodge in the esophagus and cause ulcera-
Kaon-Cl	Sugar-coated: 500 mg (6.67 mEq) in wax matrix	tions in cardiac patients who have esophageal compression due to en-
Kaon	Sugar-coated: 5 mEq potassium gluconate	larged left atrium. In patients with esophageal stasis or obstruction, use liquid form.
Parenteral (available in ampules, syringes, and vials) Potassium chloride	10 mEq/10 ml 10 mEq/15 ml 20 mEq/10 ml◇ 20 mEq/20 ml 30 mEq/10 ml 30 mEq/12.5 ml 30 mEq/15 ml 30 mEq/20 ml 40 mEq/12.5 ml 40 mEq/20 ml◇ 60 mEq/30 ml 90 mEq/30 ml	• Always administer slowly as *dilute solutions* (not to exceed 80 mEq/L); do not exceed 20 mEq/hour. Do not exceed 150 mEq/day in adults; 3 mEq/kg in children. • EKG monitoring best indicates tissue potassium levels. Also monitor plasma potassium levels. Never use until urine flow is established. • Don't administer to any patient with acute dehydration or severe renal impairment.
Potassium acetate (ampules or vials)	40 mEq/20 ml 50 mEq/20 ml 90 mEq/30 ml	• Observe for pain and redness at injection site.

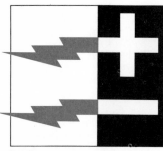

Profile on potassium
Normal plasma value:
3.5 to 5.0 mEq/liter

potassium deficit (hypokalemia) especially when:

• *aldosteronism (primary or secondary) and Cushing's syndrome* excessively stimulate the sodium/potassium exchange mechanism in the kidney. This causes the kidney to spill potassium. Remember that treatment with adrenal steroids provokes aldosteronism with the same effect

• *renal disease,* such as renal tubular acidosis, increases urinary potassium loss either by defective reabsorption or accelerated excretion (the mechanism is not known)

• *congestive heart failure* increases aldosterone levels

• *potent diuretics* (mercurials, thiazides, furosemide [Lasix], ethacrynic acid [Edecrin] and acetazolamide [Diamox]) stimulate potassium loss

• *drainage or suction of gastric contents* removes large quantities of potassium that exist normally in gastric secretions

• *prolonged vomiting* loses gastric juices which usually contain a concentration of potassium somewhat greater than that of plasma

• *diarrhea* loses fluid rich in potassium.

So, look for potassium depletion in patients with any unusual losses of body fluid, or renal or adrenal impairment. And remember to look for it even among patients seemingly not very ill. Among the seriously ill, many things can cause serious loss of potassium, including congestive heart failure, liver disease, the aftereffects of major surgery, starvation, and gastric suctioning. Expect the most pronounced depletion in connection with potent diuretics (except potassium-sparing triamterene [Dyrenium] and spironolactone [Aldactone]). Also, beware of routine infusion of potassium-free saline or dextrose. These can lower the body potassium stores to dangerous levels.

Potassium stores hard to measure
Hypokalemia can exist solely in the plasma, or it can exist in both plasma and cells. Sometimes in patients with cellular deficit, plasma levels may remain deceptively high before they drop to reflect the true condition. The serum test tells plasma potassium levels. But only the clinical history and physical examination tell much about storage levels. Acute shortages of potassium can be tolerated fairly well, but prolonged deficit brings pathologic changes in the heart and kidney.

In nursing, you watch for severe hypokalemia because it may cause ventricular fibrillation, respiratory paralysis, and cardiac arrest. For a patient on digitalis, a sharp drop in serum potassium can be fatal. Remember that many medical situations — whether apparently mild or obviously severe — can lead to such catastrophic depletion, and depletion can develop gradually or abruptly. Also remember that hypokalemia rarely occurs without a concomitant alkalosis. If the plasma concentration of potassium drops, the kidneys start excreting hydrogen ions instead of potassium to fill their electrochemical needs. Conversely, if alkalosis is already present, the kidneys will try to conserve hydrogen and will excrete potassium.

Paradoxically, either a very high or low potassium level may lead to the same neuromuscular effect; muscle weakness and flaccid paralysis. That's because either state creates an ionic imbalance in the nerve and muscle excitation process. For other symptoms of hypo- and hyperkalemia, see pp. 86-87. Fortunately, we can make early diagnosis of both states of imbalance by electrocardiography.

Correcting hypokalemia

In most patients you can correct hypokalemia easily with oral replacement (K-Lor, Kay Ciel, and others) and increased intake of potassium-rich foods. However, if the deficit is causing severe symptoms, parenteral replacement is in order. For example, you can rapidly correct the flaccid paralysis of hypokalemia if the kidneys are excreting at least 120 ml urine per hour. How? By giving a 2-hour infusion of KCl (as much as 40 mEq of potassium) in 5% dextrose in water.

When giving parenteral potassium replacement, do not infuse more than 20 mEq per hour and watch for local complications:

Irritation — Intravenous potassium can greatly irritate the patient's veins, especially if the concentration is high — more than 30 to 40 mEq/L in 500 ml of fluid. The patient may complain of a burning sensation at the I.V. site or even traveling up the entire venous branch proximal to the infusion site. With the doctor's permission, relieve such discomfort by:

- applying an icebag
- giving mild sedation, or
- anesthetizing temporarily with a small amount of procaine in the I.V. site (flashball).

Treatment for hyperkalemia may include:

- *Cation exchange resin* — (polystyrene sulfonate/Kayexalate) binds and eliminates potassium via the bowel. It can be given orally, rectally, or by nasogastric tube. A common mixture is 50 g of resin suspended in 50 ml of 70% Sorbitol and 100 ml of H_2O.
- *NaHCO_3* — intravenous infusion of 44 to 132 mEq NaHCO$_3$ added to 1 L 5% dextrose in water. NaHCO$_3$ rapidly lowers plasma potassium levels by alkalinization of plasma which causes a shift of K^+ in urine. The beneficial effect is also partly due to the dilution of the plasma K^+ by administration of a hypertonic sodium solution (i.e., 7.5% NaHCO$_3$).
- *Calcium salts* — by slow I.V. infusion of 4.5 mEq to 13.5 mEq of 10% calcium gluconate under EKG monitoring. Calcium does not alter plasma potassium levels but acts on the neuromuscular membranes and antagonizes the cardiotoxicity of hyperkalemia (when EKG shows broad QRS complexes or absent P waves). The rate of calcium infusion should not exceed 1.5 mEq/min; the total daily infusion in adults should not exceed 70 mEq. The effects of calcium infusion are rapid but transient.
- *Glucose and insulin* — by I.V. infusion of 500 ml of 10% dextrose in water and 10 units of regular insulin over 30 minutes. This infusion is followed by a slower one of just dextrose in water.
- *Dialysis* (hemo- or peritoneal dialysis) effectively removes potassium; but these methods are relatively slow compared to other treatments. Dialysis is rarely required for treating electrolyte imbalance except in patients with renal failure.

POTASSIUM IMBALANCES

Hyperkalemia

IN PATIENTS WITH:

Renal failure (prevents normal Na/K exchange)

Hemorrhagic shock: In hemorrhagic shock and acute renal failure — during severe hemorrhage and ensuing hypovolemia, the body tries to maintain blood pressure and blood volume against all odds. If hemorrhage continues, hypotension will compromise renal blood flow, and glomerular filtration rate will decrease. But now potassium released from the damaged cells into the extracellular fluid is accumulating while developing oliguria and anuria threaten renal shutdown.

Addison's disease (absence of aldosterone allows heavy excretion of sodium and water and consequent build-up of potassium)

Excessive K in intravenous therapy

Disorders with massive cell damage:
● burns
● crushing injury: disrupted cells release intracellular potassium into the plasma. Intracellular K levels can reach at least 50 times those of blood, and urinary excretion is apt to be diminished at such a time.
● myocardial infarction: heart muscle cells damaged by coronary occlusion immediately release potassium into nearby blood vessels, causing localized hyperkalemia. At a time when the heart muscle is already vulnerable to arrhythmia, excess plasma potassium may be a dire threat. The excess plasma cations lower the electric potential between beating and resting and reduce the muscle's action and potential. Repolarization speeds up. Ventricular contraction weakens. If hyperkalemia altogether prevents the ionic shift needed to conduct the electric impulse, the heart may simply stop in diastole. Look for EKG abnormalities superimposed on the abnormal Q waves, and S-T segment elevation of the EKG pattern coming from the infarct.

EXPECT THESE SYMPTOMS:
weakness
malaise
nausea
intestinal colic
diarrhea
muscle irritability
flaccid paralysis
oliguria
EKG changes diagnostic

The highs
When your patient's serum potassium level is above normal, expect the following EKG changes.

■■■ Normal   ▨▨▨ Abnormal

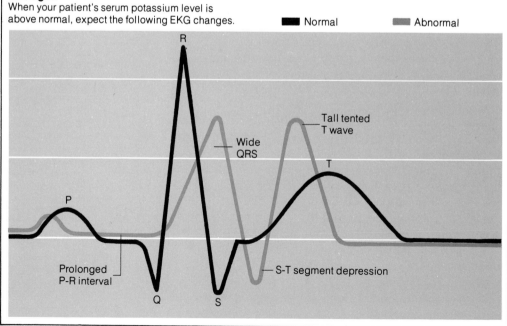

TAKE THESE ACTIONS:

Watch for early symptoms in patients at risk

Watch lab data for serum K higher than 6.0 mEq/L

Monitor EKG

Limit oral intake of potassium and protein

Encourage urinary output (increase fluid intake)

Give NaHCO₃, calcium salts, or glucose and insulin, as ordered

Assist doctor in removing excess K by:
- cation exchange resin (Kayexalate)*
- peritoneal dialysis
- hemodialysis

*In renal shutdown, carefully measure amount of water used in this treatment.

Hypokalemia

IN PATIENTS WITH:

Loss of body fluids

- diuretics (except spironolactone and triamterene)
- prolonged vomiting/diarrhea
- excessive sweating
- excessive lactation
- ulcerative colitis
- laxative habit
- gastric drainage or suction

Adrenal disorders
- aldosteronism
- Cushing's syndrome
- adrenal steroid therapy
- stress (mental or physical)

Congestive heart failure

Villous adenoma of rectum

Licorice candy addiction (glyceric acid has aldosterone-like effect)

EXPECT THESE SYMPTOMS:

Disturbed muscle function
- gastrointestinal
- skeletal
- cardiac

Decreased reflexes

Muscular irritability or weakness

Speech changes (reflect partial muscle paralysis)

Rapid, weak, irregular pulse

Drop in blood pressure

Abdominal distention, flatulence, vomiting, and paralytic ileus

EKG changes diagnostic

TAKE THESE ACTIONS:

Maintain accurate intake/output records

Monitor pulse and EKG

Watch for early symptoms, especially muscle weakness and fatigue

Watch for serum K below 3.5 mEq/L

Watch for these signs of metabolic alkalosis: nausea, vomiting and diarrhea followed by mental confusion and irritability

Give K replacement as ordered.

The lows
When your patient's serum potassium level is below normal, expect the following EKG changes. ■ Normal ■ Abnormal

R

P

Q S

T

Flattened T wave

U wave

S-T segment depression

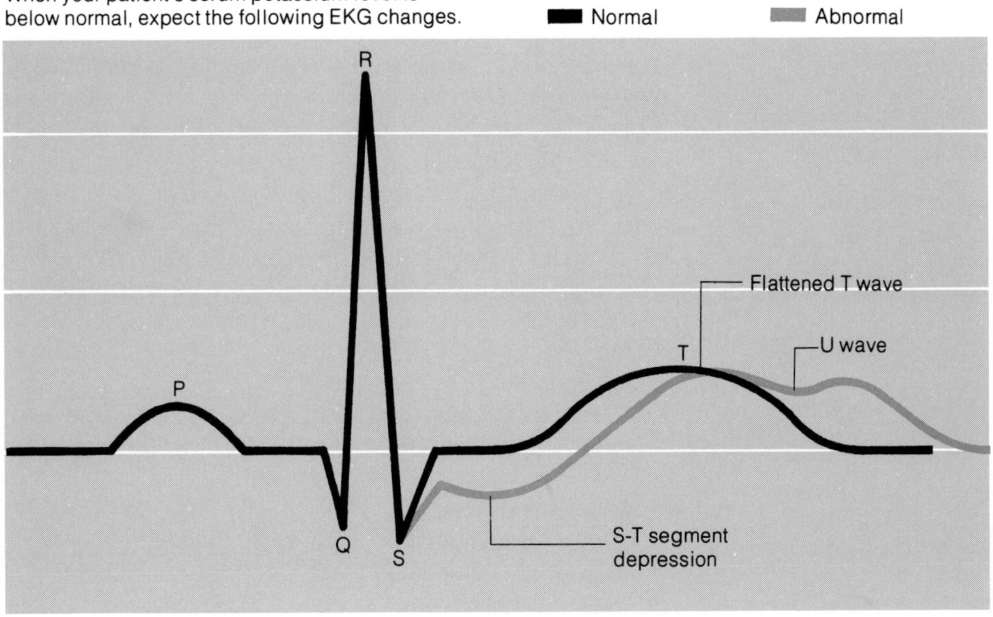

Never give potassium or other electrolytes subcutaneously or intramuscularly.

Phlebitis — Watch for chemical phlebitis, especially in critically ill patients unable to communicate pain. Carefully inspect the site for redness or heat, and report any evidence of phlebitis promptly. If it's very severe, you could change the site of infusion or suggest a more dilute solution. Severe phlebitis usually requires treatment with warm soaks.

Special caution! I.V. replacement

A serious threat to any patient on I.V. therapy is an error in judgment about adding potassium to circulating fluid. Critically high levels of potassium can accumulate rapidly. When giving potassium intravenously — and give it only after urine flow has been established to be sure the kidneys can regulate it — infuse potassium no faster than 15 to 20 mEq/L per hour, and no more concentrated than 40 to 80 mEq/L of fluid. If laboratory reports show serum levels of potassium as high as 6 mEq/L, the patient needs treatment for hyperkalemia. Otherwise, he may develop ventricular fibrillation.

In the seriously ill patient, whose homeostasis is already seriously compromised, hyperkalemia can develop rapidly. If so, he'll need help quickly. To give such help, watch for general weakness, malaise, nausea, intestinal colic, and diarrhea resulting from the body's attempts to eliminate surplus potassium. As serum potassium rises, the patient may progress to muscle irritability, flaccid paralysis, oliguria (to conserve the dwindling water stores) and even anuria. But early stages of hyperkalemia (like *hypo*kalemia) are best detected by the electrocardiographic pattern (see pages 86 and 87). Watch for these telltale changes in patients likely to accumulate excessive potassium levels — those with kidney and adrenal failure or impairment, and with severe injuries.

Expect hyperkalemia

You can expect hyperkalemia in situations that allow heavy excretion of sodium; release of intracellular potassium stores; and decreased excretion of potassium:
- Addison's disease
- hemorrhagic shock and acute renal failure
- massive crushing injury, and
- myocardial infarction.

Sodium
CONTROLLER OF FLUID VOLUME

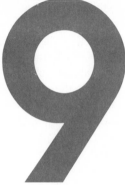

BY LAWRENCE WOLFE, BSc

YOUR PATIENT'S LAB REPORT just came in and shows a low serum sodium. Do you know how to decide if it reflects a real or apparent sodium deficit? Actually, this patient's total body sodium could be high, low, or normal. Do you know what other clinical features to look for to decide which it is? Each of these states produces a particular disorder and each needs its own special treatment. More than any other electrolyte, sodium influences the distribution of body water. It also helps maintain acid-base balance and neuromuscular function. Wherever you practice nursing, you need to know how to recognize the several kinds of sodium imbalance and know what to do about them.

Why is sodium important?
Sodium is the most abundant cation in extracellular fluid. At its normal concentration, 136 to 145 mEq/L, it supplies almost 90% of the total cations. Sodium affects many vital functions and is mainly responsible for the osmotic pressure of the extracellular fluid. This is partly because of its prevalence in the body and partly because it does not easily cross the cell membrane.

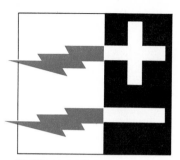

Profile on sodium
Normal plasma value:
136 to 145 mEq/liter

It's nearly impossible to discuss body sodium without also mentioning water. Indeed sodium and water are so inseparable that talking of one without the other is like talking of Laurel without Hardy. The sodium concentration of the extracellular fluid profoundly influences the kidney's regulation of the body's water and electrolyte status. For example, when sodium concentration falls, the kidneys promote water excretion under the influence of aldosterone and other stimuli; when sodium concentration rises, the release of ADH causes the kidneys to retain more water and subsequently dilute the sodium to normal levels.

Sodium promotes the irritability of nerve and muscle tissue and the conduction of nerve impulses and influences the body's vital acid-base balance.

Generally, the body's regulatory mechanisms hold the sodium-water relationship within normal limits. But illness can throw this relationship severely out of balance.

First, hyponatremia

Hyponatremia simply means that the amount of sodium in the extracellular compartment is deficient as compared to the amount of water. Several things can cause this deficiency:

• *Water intoxication* occurs when a patient continues normal, or above normal, intake of water despite inability, or decreased ability to excrete it. Such intoxications may be mild, moderate, or severe. Severe hyponatremia (when serum sodium level is 115 mEq/L or less) usually causes confusion, clouded sensorium, muscle twitching, or sometimes even grand mal seizures.

Treatment of choice is to restrict water intake, *not* to give hypertonic saline. Only in extremely rare cases of severe and symptomatic hyponatremia (when Na^+ is below 110 mEq/L) is treatment with 3% or 5% saline indicated. Then it's only to bring the patient back to a non-symptomatic state, not to replace the sodium deficit. This treatment is quite dangerous; it can easily lead to disastrous circulatory overload.

• *Dilutional hyponatremia* occurs with expansion of total body water, i.e. CHF, renal failure, cirrhosis. This condition is treated by restricting water intake. Only if severe symptoms of hyponatremia occur is saline required. Remember that in this condition there is increased total body sodium, even though serum levels are low.

• *SIADH (sydrome of inappropriate secretion of ADH)* can be caused by some malignant tumors, cerebral disorders, or cirrhosis. The resulting hyponatremia is dilutional, a result of water retention. Once again, the best treatment is water restriction. Water intake should be restricted to less than combined sensible and insensible losses until the serum sodium concentration returns to normal. After that, water can be given in amounts equal to sensible and insensible losses. Another treatment for SIADH is to administer furosemide (Lasix) IV. (The urine is collected and measured for Na^+ and K^+ content. The Na^+ and K^+ losses are replaced hourly, using 3% saline with added KCl.) This method requires much care and is inconvenient from everyone's point of view, but it can correct severe hyponatremia within hours.

• *True hyponatremia* (low body sodium), occurs as a result of extra-renal salt loss. Some causes: burns, diarrhea, prolonged vomiting, treatment with diuretics (especially in patients whose sodium is restricted), adrenal insufficiency, drainage from fistulas, and salt-losing renal disorders. Because of such loss, the patient cannot maintain a normal volume of extracellular fluid and shows signs of dehydration, such as loss of skin turgor. At the same time, as all his extracellular compartments shrink, the patient develops clinical signs of hypovolemia (tachycardia, hypotension, orthostatic hypotension, azotemia, and oliguria). These changes, typical of low extracellular fluid volume, confirm the diagnosis of low body sodium.

• Hyperlipidemia, hypoproteinemia, and hyperglycemia can contribute to false, *hypertonic hyponatremias*. At first glance, this seems a contradiction. How can you have both hyponatremia and hypertonic extracellular fluid? If you recall the formula for calculating osmolality (see Chapter 1), you can see that the sodium term is the most important only if you plug in *normal* values for all terms. However, if you substitute values for a patient with uncontrolled diabetes and a high blood sugar (say, 280 mg/100 ml), then the formula looks different. Remember that osmolality is entirely dependent on the total number of particles in solution. If we greatly increase one of the terms in the equation, in this case glucose, osmolality of the extracellular fluid increases appreciably. As osmolality rises, it pulls water from the intracellular compartments in an attempt to even out the concentration difference. This addi-

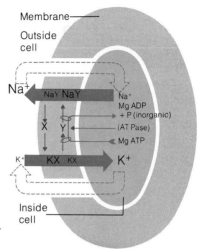

The sodium pump
The processes of depolarization and repolarization (see page 23) cause sodium to diffuse into the cells and potassium to diffuse out of the cells, disrupting the ionic balance. Although sodium and potassium don't easily penetrate the cell membrane, in combination with a carrier they can become soluble in the lipoprotein membrane and can be transported across to their original compartments.

It is thought that a single carrier transports both ions. This carrier is called Y when it has an affinity for sodium and X after it undergoes a chemical transformation which changes its affinity, allowing it to combine with potassium. Adenosine triphosphate (ATP) and ATPase provide the energy needed for this transformation as well as for splitting the cations from the carrier at the appropriate moment. The entire cycle goes on indefinitely and is referred to as the sodium pump. It helps transmit neuromuscular impulses, stimulate glandular secretions, and prevent cellular swelling.

Sodium signs and symptoms
Since sodium is the predominant extracellular cation, a sodium imbalance has a profound effect on the body. Here's a handy list of signs and symptoms you will see in patients suffering from sodium excess or deficit:
HYPERNATREMIA
Symptoms
  Thirst
Signs
  Dry sticky membranes
  Flushed skin
  Fever
  Rough dry tongue
  Oliguria
  Plasma osmolality > 1.5 mOsm/L
  Urine SG > 1.015 if water loss is
    nonrenal
  Urine SG < 1.010 if diabetes
    insipidus, diuretic phase of
    acute tubular necrosis
  Serum sodium > 145mEq/L
HYPONATREMIA
Symptoms
  Weakness, apathy, lassitude
  Irritability, apprehension
  Headaches
Signs
  Weight loss, or edema and
    weight gain
  Hypotension
  Decreased skin turgor
  Tremors and convulsions
  Serum sodium < 135 mEq/L
  Serum osmolality: decreased
    with retention; increased with
    diuresis
  Urine SG < 1.010 with diuresis;
  >1.010 with water retention

tional water dilutes the concentration of extracellular electrolytes, including sodium. Thus we have hyponatremia in a hypertonic extracellular fluid due to high glucose concentration.

Treatment, of course, aims to remove the excess glucose molecules. Incidentally, since one of the homeostatic mechanisms for getting rid of hypertonicity is excretion of sodium, treatment of such a diabetic initially includes I.V. sodium replacement with infusion of 0.9% saline.

• *Starvation hyponatremia* is a special form of sodium deficit that occurs in patients with cancer, in imprudent dieters, and in other persons who have been deprived of food for a long time. Many patients with chronic debilitating disease have no clinical symptoms of dehydration or edema and no apparent disturbance of water metabolism, yet their sodium levels are abnormally low. This condition appears to result from starvation; it is common in any patient who's lost more than 15% of body weight. Such a patient looks wasted, his skin turgor is poor, he is apt to be anemic, and his albumin levels are low. His serum concentration may be as low as 125 to 133 mEq/L. This hypotonicity seems unaffected by treatment with salt, and thus differs from simple sodium depletion. And, since it cannot be corrected by water restriction, it is also different from hypotonicity of water excess. Treatment of this condition *does not* include giving salt. It requires *improved nutrition*. In surgical patients with cancer (in whom such hyponatremia is common) treatment includes high-protein nutrition and blood transfusions.

Hypernatremia most dangerous
Hypernatremia and its resulting hyperosmolality, occurs when water losses exceed sodium losses or when water intake is inadequate. Very seldom does it reflect a gain in sodium (although this does happen in hyperaldosteronism). The usual cause of such hypernatremia is the excessive loss of water. In such cases it accompanies cellular and extracellular dehydration. As water is lost due to profuse sweating, diarrhea, polyuria, diabetes insipidus or mellitus, and high-protein tube feedings, the extracellular fluid becomes hypertonic. This draws water from the intracellular compartments with the result that both compartments, the intracellular and extracellular, contain excess sodium relative to volume of water.

Some Sodium Supplements

PRODUCT	AMOUNT OF SODIUM SUPPLIED	NURSING TIPS
Tablets Sodium chloride	300 mg, 500 mg, 600 mg, 650 mg, 1 g, 2.25 g, 2.5 g Enteric coated: 1 g	• Enteric coated tablets must not be crushed, chewed or dissolved
Sodium chloride with dextrose	455 mg sodium chloride and 195 mg dextrose (also with Vitamin B_1)	
Thermotabs	450 mg sodium chloride, 30 mg potassium chloride, 18 mg calcium carbonate, 200 mg dextrose	
Oral solution Moyer's solution	Sodium chloride 0.3% and sodium bicarbonate 0.15%	• Especially useful to replace fluids after burns and injuries
Parenteral Sodium chloride	0.45% solution (0.45 gram/100 ml) 0.9% solution (0.9 gram/100 ml) 3% solution (3 grams/100 ml) 5% solution (5 grams/100 ml)	• Watch for signs of electrolyte imbalance: water retention, edema, and aggravation of hypokalemia, or acidosis. Hypertonic solutions 3% and 5% can cause increased venous pressure. Administer cautiously in small quantities by slow I.V.
Sodium bicarbonate◇	4.2% (500 mEq/L) in 10 ml 5% (595 mEq/L) in 500 ml 7.5% (892 mEq/L) in 50 ml 8.4% (1000 mEq/L) in 50 ml and 10 ml.	• In infants, don't exceed 8 mEq/kg/day to avoid hypernatremia, decreased cerebrospinal fluid pressure, and intracranial hemorrhage.
Neut	4% (480 mEq/L) in 50 ml	• Usually given rapidly during cardiac arrest. (In less urgent metabolic acidosis, infuse hypertonic $NaHCO_3$ at 2 to 5 mEq/kg over 4 to 8 hours to avoid overcorrection to alkalosis.
Ringer's lactate solution	130 mEq/L of sodium chloride and 27 mEq/L of sodium lactate (plus potassium and calcium)	• Give sodium solutions cautiously to patients with CHF, kidney dysfunction, or circulatory insufficiency.

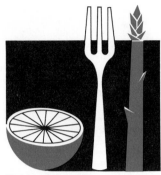

Not worth the salt
Instruct your edematous patient to
avoid all foods high in sodium,
which include the following:
- salted "snack" foods such as
  potato chips, peanuts;
- canned soups and vegetables;
- dried fruits;
- delicatessen foods, especially
  lox;
- prepared "pre-portion" foods
  such as TV dinners;
- preserved meat (such as hot
  dogs) and luncheon meats;
- cheeses of all kinds (including
  cottage);
- anything preserved in brine,
  such as olives, pickles, and
  sauerkraut.

Hypernatremia also follows inadequate water intake mainly in patients with hypothalamic lesions or coma. In *any* patient who cannot ask for or obtain water, think of hypernatremia. It's a possible complication in any condition in which more water is lost than electrolytes. It's a common complication in tracheobronchitis, in which excessive water is lost from the lungs due to fever and deep rapid breathing and in profuse watery diarrhea when treatment is inadequate. Infants with severe diarrhea are especially vulnerable to hypernatremia (with high mortality — about 50%). So are unconscious patients and others who cannot ask for or drink water.

Salt intoxication

Rarely, hypernatremia does follow a gain in sodium, not loss of water. If a large quantity of sodium is added to the extracellular fluid, and the addition takes place abruptly, the consequences can be devastating. Water pours out of cells and overloads the interstitial and vascular compartments. This usually happens as an unfortunate side effect of treatment. For example, hypertonic sodium bicarbonate (usually 7.5% sodium bicarbonate) is often given in large quantities to treat cardiac arrest or lactic acidosis; and, hypertonic sodium chloride is used to induce abortion. The resulting abrupt change in extracellular fluid osmolality induces a massive redistribution of body water. In an extreme case, it can cause immediate convulsions and pulmonary edema.

Clinical findings in sodium excess include dry, sticky, mucous membranes; flushed skin; intense thirst; and rough dry tongue. Body tissues are firm since water from the cellular fluid, following the law of osmosis, flows into the more concentrated extracellular fluid. The patient may have oliguria, anuria, and fever. He may appear manic, agitated and restless; the patient may develop convulsions. The plasma sodium is usually above 147 mEq/L — but may range higher. Plasma chloride is above 106 mEq/L, and specific gravity of urine is above 1.030.

The treatment for hypernatremia is to give *salt-free solutions*. Water may be given orally if the serum sodium concentration is below about 150 to 160 mEq/L. It is usual practice to give salt-free solutions, such as 5% dextrose in water, until the sodium level returns to normal and then switch over to 0.45% saline sodium to avoid overcorrection to deficit.

Aldosterone and certain drugs

Aldosterone conserves sodium by inhibiting its excretion; it promotes potassium excretion at the level of the distal tubule. How this happens is clear if you remember that ions are electrically charged particles and that, in nature, all things tend to seek an equilibrium. Remember too, that the glomerular filtrate is a solution of many ions, such as the positively charged hydrogen, sodium, and potassium ions and the negatively charged chloride, phosphate, and bicarbonate ions. This solution is electrically neutral if neither a (+) or (−) charge exists. So, if aldosterone conserves sodium ions, which are positively charged, then a negative electrical charge is left in the filtrate. This sets up an electrical pressure for some positively charged ions to replace the sodium ions. Two such ions are available, potassium and hydrogen. But hydrogen is already present in the filtrate at a greater concentration than in the tubular epithelial cells. So potassium diffuses into the filtrate to provide electrical neutralization and gets excreted. Next, the reabsorbed sodium ions leave the tubular epithelial cells and go into the renal capillary circulation. Water follows the sodium (by osmotic effect). The end result is an expanded extracellular fluid volume.

Other drugs that influence sodium concentration or metabolism include: all diuretics, chlorpropamide (Diabinese), vasopressin (Pitressin), antihypertensive agents, and corticosteroids. Though each kind of diuretic has a different site of action in the tubule, they all tend to promote excretion of sodium by inhibiting reabsorption.

By contrast, chlorpropamide, a sulfonylurea hypoglycemic agent, appears to cause an impairment of free water excretion, causing hyponatremia by way of water intoxication. It seems to mimic and potentiate antidiuretic hormone (ADH or vasopressin). The hypolipemic agent, clofibrate (Atromid-S), has similar effects. Consequently, these drugs are sometimes used to treat diabetes insipidus. ADH or vasopressin, of course, has the same effect.

Various antihypertensive agents, among them, methyldopa (Aldomet), hydralazine (Apresoline), clonidine (Catapres), and reserpine (Serpasil), tend to cause sodium and water retention, with progressive loss of antihypertensive effect that generally resists increased dosage. For this reason, diuretics are usually prescribed along with antihypertensive drugs. In

Sodium content of commonly used OTC products

ANTACIDS/ANTIFLATULANTS

Riopan-Magaldrate	0.7 mg/tsp
Maalox and	
Maalox Plus	2.5 mg/tsp
Gaviscon	0.8 mEq/tsp
Alka-Seltzer;	
Bisodol	276 mg/tsp

LAXATIVES/STOOL SOFTENERS

Surfak	none
Metamucil	negligible
Metamucil (packets)	high
Konsyl	none
Feen-a mint	none
Dulcolax Suppositories	none
Fletcher's Castoria	none
Haley's M-O	high
Milk of Magnesia	high
Fleet's	high
Senokot	high
Colace	negligible

COUGH PREPARATIONS

Robitussin	none
Robitussin A-C and DM	none
Silence is Golden	none
Romilar	none
Congespirin	none
Coricidin and Coricidin D	none
Vicks' Formula 44	none

WEIGHT CONTROL

Sweeta	none

addition to counteracting sodium retention, they themselves have mild antihypertensive effects. In many patients, a diuretic is all that is needed to control hypertension.

Corticosteroids such as fludrocortisone (Florinef) promote sodium retention and potassium excretion activity (mineralocorticoid activity).

Given these facts about sodium, can you identify the imbalance in Jeff Crandall? A 22-year-old college student, Jeff was hospitalized after an automobile accident in which he suffered head trauma. After an emergency craniotomy, he remained comatose. His treatment included I.V. fluid (5% dextrose in water, 1000 ml/24 hours); enteral feeding (EF) to provide nitrogen and calories; and prophylactic ampicillin (1 g I.V. q 4h). He developed diarrhea on the 2nd postoperative day; by the 4th day, his serum sodium had fallen to 120 mEq/L. The total fluid volume he received each day was about 2000 ml (roughly half of this was supplied by the EF). His intake and output nearly matched (but output was slightly greater due to the diarrhea). However, his sodium intake per 24 hours was found to be only 10 mEq/L.

Let's review the significant facts about Jeff. He was comatose; total I.V. intake 2000 ml/day; had diarrhea; intake almost equals output, with output slightly greater; and Na^+ content of enteral feeding low. With these facts alone you can suspect that Jeff was hyponatremic. And that diarrhea plus inadequate sodium replacement were causing his hyponatremia. Postoperative hyponatremia is usually due to the dilutional effect of excessive water intake or to ADH/aldosterone imbalance. Its usual treatment is water restriction. But in this patient water restriction would have been clearly inappropriate. His treatment began with changing his intravenous infusion to 5% dextrose in 0.45% normal saline. His serum sodium returned to normal (136 mEq/L) within 2 days.

Even though patients who cannot ask for water often develop *hyper*natremia, Jeff developed *hypo*natremia. In this case, it was more helpful to remember that the patient who is restricted to parenteral feedings must receive some salt in them, or he will become hyponatremic.

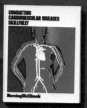
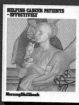
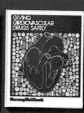
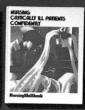
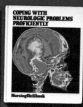
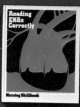
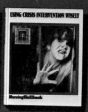
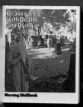
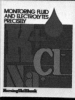
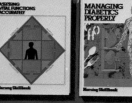
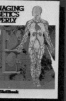
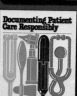
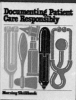
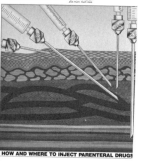

Choose one of these important books as your introductory volume when you join the NURSING SKILLBOOK series...the most comprehensive reference series ever published for nurses.

• Using Crisis Intervention Wisely • Coping With Neurologic Problems Proficiently • Managing Diabetics Properly • Helping Cancer Patients Effectively • Documenting Patient Care Responsibly • Monitoring Fluid and Electrolytes Precisely • Giving Cardiovascular Drugs Safely • Assessing Vital Functions Accurately • Nursing Critically Ill Patients Confidently • Giving Emergency Care Competently • Reading EKGs Correctly • Combatting Cardiovascular Diseases Skillfully • Dealing with Death and Dying

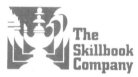

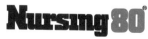

Calcium
THE DURABLE ELECTROLYTE

10

BY RUSSEL THOMAS, BSc

SERUM CALCIUM IMBALANCE is a real medical emergency. As deficit, it produces tetany and seizures; as excess, it produces lethargy, dehydration, cardiac arrhythmia and even coma. You can handle such emergencies better — and sometimes prevent them — if you know: how the body balances calcium; how to recognize calcium imbalance; what causes it; and how to treat it.

Calcium: Most abundant
The human body contains about 1200 grams of calcium, of which about 99% is tied up in bone. This bone calcium exists mainly as insoluble crystals, which gives bone its hardness and durability. Bone calcium is physiologically inactive. Only the remaining 1% of the total body calcium found in the soft tissues and serum is the active amount we deal with in patients with calcium imbalance.

Three things influence the serum calcium balance: the deposition and resorption of bone; the absorption of calcium from the gastrointestinal tract; and the excretion of calcium in the urine and feces. First and most important is the *deposition and resorption of bone*. Even though bone calcium is

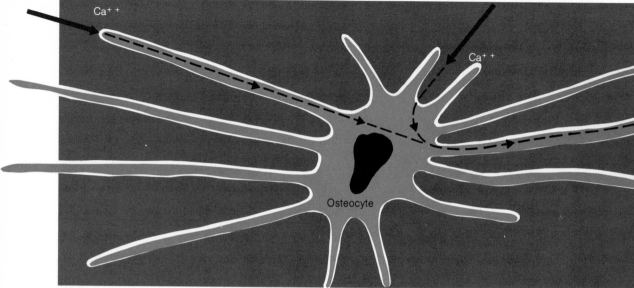

physiologically inactive, calcium does exchange between the bone and serum. This exchange is carried on by the cellular components of bone, the osteocytes. These cells may be either osteoblasts (which deposit calcium and form new bone) or osteoclasts (which move calcium from bone into serum). Parathyroid hormone (PTH) and large doses of vitamin D stimulate these cells to transfer calcium from the bones to raise the serum calcium level. In the other direction, the hormone, calcitonin, and high levels of phosphate stimulate them to transfer calcium from the serum into the bones to *lower* calcium level.

The *absorption of calcium* from the gastrointestinal tract depends mainly, of course, on the dietary intake. Dietary vitamin D promotes calcium absorption through the intestine; phosphates inhibit it. Phosphates, vitamin D, and parathyroid hormone regulate calcium excretion in the urine and feces. Parathyroid hormone, vitamin D, and phosphates all work together to both increase and decrease the serum calcium. When these elements are normal, calcium excretion remains fairly constant.

Evaluate serum calcium

The value we usually use for discussing a patient's calcium requirements is the serum calcium level. The normal range for serum calcium is 8.8 to 10.5 mg per 100 ml. But the serum calcium level does not tell the whole story and is useful only if you know how to interpret it. About half (56%) of the serum calcium is bound to plasma proteins. This means it's chemically inactive. When we speak of the active serum calcium we mean only the ionized (non-protein bound) portion. This physiological relationship of calcium to serum protein means that any change in the serum protein (as often occurs in renal disease), changes the total serum calcium. This change amounts to about 0.8 mg/100 ml of calcium for each 1 g/100 ml change in protein (albumin).

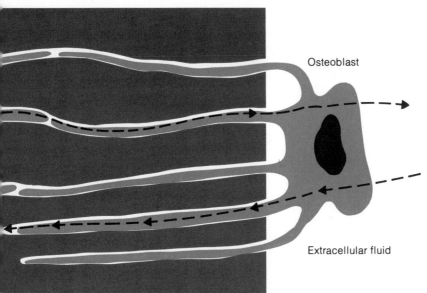

Osteoblast

Extracellular fluid

Deposits and returns
Under healthy conditions, calcium shifts naturally in and out of the bones, a process which allows for bone building as well as the immediate correction of any deviation in serum calcium levels. Normally the withdrawal and retrieval of calcium balance one another.

This is how it all works: Mature bone cells called osteocytes withdraw calcium from the serum and bone. The osteocytes transport calcium to an osteoblast, an immature bone cell. The osteoblast pumps the calcium back into the extracellular fluid and then retrieves it again, depositing it back into the bone.

Let's run through a sample calculation to see how this works. If a patient has a serum calcium of 9.0 mg/100 ml and a serum albumin of 4 g/100 ml (normal is 3.5 to 5 g/100 ml), both his calcium and albumin values are in the normal range. At a later time, the patient's serum calcium is still 9.0 mg/100 ml but his albumin has dropped to 1 g/100 ml. Is his calcium still normal? Work it out thus: Because albumin has dropped by 3 g/100 ml, multiply 3 times 0.8. This equals 2.4 mg/100 ml of calcium. When you add this 2.4 to his serum calcium 9.0, the corrected serum calcium is 11.4 mg/100 ml — definitely excessive. So, this patient is hypercalcemic, even though the lab reports a "normal" value for serum calcium. This is the method doctors use to interpret a serum calcium value, and you should know about it.

Recognize hypocalcemia
Hypocalcemia is relatively rare, but you will meet it occasionally, especially in hospitalized patients. Hypocalcemia may result from hypoparathyroidism, vitamin D deficiency, pancreatitis, magnesium deficiency, or chronic laxative ingestion. It may also follow surgery involving the parathyroid or thyroid glands. The symptoms of hypocalcemia include perioral paresthesias, twitching, carpopedal spasm, tetany and seizures, and may include cardiac arrhythmias. When hypocalcemia is severe, it needs immediate treatment.

Watch for hypocalcemia especially in patients recovering from surgery involving the parathyroids or thyroid. In such patients, diminished parathyroid hormone upsets the calcium balance. The serum calcium may drop precipitously, even resulting in tetany or seizures. For this reason, you are often required to keep calcium gluconate ampules at the bedside after such surgery. Patients receiving hemodialysis or hyperalimentation also risk calcium deficiency, so their management should always include regular laboratory tests for serum calcium.

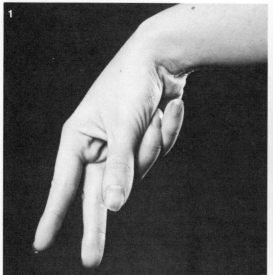

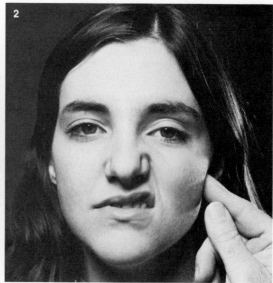

Seek a sign

A calcium deficit causes the membranes of nerve fibers to become partially charged. This increased irritability produces the transmission of repetitive and uncontrolled impulses and muscular spasms such as Trousseau's sign and Chvostek's sign.

Trousseau's sign (Figure 1), found in latent tetany, is a carpopedal spasm that may occur spontaneously or can even be stimulated by the application of a blood pressure cuff. The patient's thumb adducts and his phalangeal joints extend, as shown.

You can induce Chvostek's sign (Figure 2) in a patient with hypocalcemia by tapping the facial nerve adjacent to the ear. This will produce a muscle contraction that causes the patient's upper lip to twitch as shown.

Treatment of acute hypocalcemia requires the intravenous administration of a calcium salt, usually calcium gluconate. The usual dosage is 10 to 20 ml of a 10% solution. This may be given quickly in a small volume of 5% dextrose or may be given cautiously by I.V. push into a large vein. An additional dose, usually 20 to 30 ml, is then given more slowly in a liter of 5% dextrose. Do not use saline to infuse calcium supplements because it may encourage calcium loss. Saline is actually used to treat hypercalcemia, as we'll see later on. Also, do not add calcium salts to I.V. solutions containing bicarbonate because they will rapidly precipitate.

The calcium ion has an effect on the myocardium that is similar to that of digitalis. So, calcium is generally not given to patients who are taking digitalis.

What about oral calcium supplements? These are used for chronic hypocalcemia, often with vitamin D. The oral dosage range for hypocalcemia is 1.5 to 3 grams of calcium per day. Remember that this amount is stated as *elemental* calcium, whereas the dosage of calcium supplements is often stated as the amount of calcium *salts*. This creates a certain amount of confusion about dosage. For example, compare calcium gluconate (9% elemental calcium) and calcium lactate (13% elemental calcium). Both are available for oral use as 600 mg tablets. But these 600 mg tablets are not equivalent, since the gluconate supplies only 54 mg of elemental calcium while the lactate supplies 78 mg. These differences can be important, especially when a patient is switched from one to the other. (See table.)

Vitamin D is a part of the treatment for chronic hypocalcemia since it facilitates absorption of calcium supplements. Dosage depends on the patient's response and usually ranges from 50,000 units to 250,000 units per day. Three forms of vitamin D are commonly used: ergocalciferol (vitamin D_2), cholecalciferol (vitamin D_3), and dihydrotachysterol. The doses of vitamin D_2 and D_3 are usually stated in units; of dihydrotachysterol, in milligrams. The latter is a synthetic form of the vitamin which is much more potent than vitamin D_2 or D_3 and is often used when a patient fails to respond satisfactorily to vitamin D_2 or D_3. Vitamin D is available as an injection for intramuscular use. High doses are sometimes used to treat tetany in hypoparathyroid patients. But for treatment of mild deficiency states, the amounts of vitamin D in most multi-vitamin preparations are adequate.

Hypercalcemia more common

The symptoms of hypercalcemia include lethargy, anorexia, nausea and vomiting, constipation, and dehydration. In hospitalized patients, these symptoms are often difficult to identify as due to hypercalcemia, since they are so common to other disease states. When hypercalcemia becomes severe (above 15 mg/100 ml) it may cause cardiac arrhythmias and coma. The many causes of hypercalcemia include primary hyperparathyroidism, parathyroid adenoma, multiple myeloma, vitamin D overdose, overuse of certain antacids, metastatic carcinomas, Paget's disease, and other skeletal diseases. Most of these conditions increase calcium mobilization from bone.

Think of treatment for hypercalcemia in two stages: the acute stage and, since the underlying problem is often a chronic disease, maintenance therapy. The first thing to do is to assure adequate hydration. This reduces the risk of renal damage and may lower the serum calcium somewhat by dilution. Rehydration is done with normal saline infusion, which is then continued to produce a saline diuresis. How much normal saline to infuse and how rapidly depends on the patient's response. But the standard dose is 1000 ml, q 4 to 6 hours.

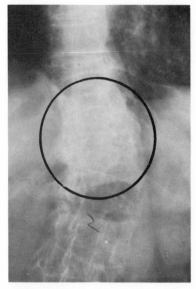

In the bones
This X-ray of an 87-year-old woman shows osteoporosis, an absolute decrease in bone tissue mass. Although experts are not sure why this degeneration occurs, they attribute the cause to defective calcium absorption in the intestines and deterioration due to aging. Some experts think that menopause or insufficient bone formation in early life causes osteoporosis.

On the X-ray you can see how the deterioration of the trabecular structure (the supporting strands of connective tissue found on the vertebrae) has decreased the radiodensity of the bones. Notice, too, the prominence of the cortical end plates and the presence of scoliosis.

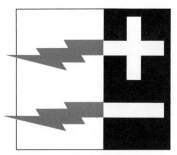

Profile on calcium
Normal plasma value:
4.5 to 5.5 mEq/liter or
8.8 to 10.5 mg/100 ml

Because the kidneys selectively reabsorb sodium, saline infusion increases calcium excretion in the urine. You need to match the rate and amount of the saline infusion to the patient's urine output, so success with this treatment depends on an accurate measure of the patient's hourly and total urine output. If saline alone does not produce adequate diuresis, furosemide (Lasix) may be given to increase urinary output and calcium excretion. Notice that the diuretics used to treat hypercalcemia are the "loop diuretics" (furosemide or ethacrynic acid [Edecrin]). Thiazide diuretics are not used because they have a different diuretic mechanism and will actually *inhibit* calcium excretion.

Phosphate lowers serum calcium by promoting deposition of calcium in bone and decreasing absorption from the GI tract. It's useful for treating both acute and chronic hypercalcemia. Phosphate is usually given orally as sodium phosphate solution (Fleet Phosphosoda) 5 ml three or four times daily. Unfortunately, this often produces diarrhea as a side effect. If the patient is unable to swallow, it may be given as phosphate-retention enemas, as it absorbs easily from the colon. For long-term management of hypercalcemia, oral phosphate is added to a low-calcium diet. Intravenous infusions of potassium or sodium phosphate are used only rarely because they may cause hypocalcemia, hypokalemia, renal damage, shock, and soft-tissue calcification, a major problem.

Corticosteroids (Cortef) and mithramycin (Mithracin) are also used for treating hypercalcemia. Corticosteroids work especially well against hypercalcemia secondary to nonparathyroid tumors. Doses of prednisone in such use range to 40 mg per day and require several days for maximal effect. Mithramycin is an anti-tumor drug which also lowers serum calcium. Its effect on serum calcium usually begins within 12 to 24 hours. Mithramycin dosage is 25 mcg/kg. It is given daily by I.V. push for 2 days. Mithramycin shares the cytotoxicities of other anti-tumor drugs: thrombocytopenia, hepatic damage and, rarely, bone-marrow depression. Although such toxicity is less prevalent in the low doses used for hypercalcemia, mithramycin is usually reserved for treating hypercalcemia due to malignancy, or when other treatment fails.

Let's review calcium imbalance as it was recognized and treated in Jim McTavish, a 53-year-old salesman.

He was admitted to the hospital because of weakness,

Some Commonly Used Calcium Supplements		
PRODUCT	AMOUNT OF CALCIUM SUPPLIED*	NURSING TIPS
Tablets Calcium gluconate◇ Calcium lactate◇	27 mg/300 mg 45 mg/500 mg 54 mg/600 mg 90 mg/1 g 39 mg/300 mg 78 mg/600 mg 84 mg/650 mg	● Well tolerated and inexpensive. Give with meals (except dairy products) because phosphorus may interfere with calcium absorption. Corticosteroids may interfere with calcium absorption. Calcium may reduce the blood levels of tetracycline; don't give within 1 hour of each other.
Liquids Neo-Calglucon syrup Calcium-Rougier◇◇	115 mg/5 ml 19 mg/ml	● Administer a.c.
Powders Calcium carbonate Calcium phosphate	400 mg/g 230 mg/g	● Less soluble than other oral forms
Parenterals Calcium chloride Calcium gluconate◇	10% solution/10 ml (270 mg) 10% solution/10 ml (90 mg)	● Very irritating. Take extreme care to avoid extravasation when you give I.V. (in cardiac arrest). Not suitable for oral use due to gastric irritation
*1 mEq elemental calcium equals 20 mg		

nausea and vomiting, and fatigue. Six months before, he was diagnosed as having multiple myeloma. On the present admission, he was cachectic and lethargic, and he complained of pain in his joints and back. He gave a history of anorexia and nausea for 4 weeks before admission. The laboratory report showed severe anemia. Some of his serum electrolyte values were: sodium, 131 mEq/L; potassium, 4.4 mEq/L; chloride, 88 mEq/L; calcium, 18.4 mg/100 ml; phosphate, 3.6 mg/100 ml; total protein, 7.7 g/100 ml; albumin, 4.1 g/100 ml; creatinine, 1.9 mg/100 ml; and BUN, 48 mg/100 ml. His EKG revealed some Q-T abnormalities and occasional PVCs. The doctor diagnosed hypercalcemia.

The patient's condition and history show dehydration as a result of anorexia and vomiting. His joint and back pain are typical of multiple myeloma and signal the presence of characteristic bone lesions. (This was confirmed by X-ray.) His calcium is very high; albumin is normal; phosphate is normal. He has EKG changes typical of hypercalcemia. All of these findings confirm hypercalcemia secondary to osteolytic lesions of multiple myeloma. This patient's lethargy and cardiac arrhythmia point to the severity of his condition and the need for immediate treatment.

An I.V. infusion of 1000 ml normal saline was begun and run over 4 hours. Four additional liters of normal saline were ordered, each to run over 4 hours. Urine output was to be monitored and the saline infusion volume matched to the urine output if greater than 250 ml/hour. Three doses of furosemide (40 mg each) were given 2 hours apart.

The lab reported his serum calcium as 16.9 mg/100 ml. His urine output after the third and fourth liters was only an additional 250 ml. The patient was having some dyspnea, suggesting fluid overload. So, the saline infusion was discontinued and a decision made to try mithramycin, 1600 mcg intravenously (25 mcg x 65 kg = 1625 mcg dose). The following day, his serum calcium was 15.4 mg/100 ml, and another dose of mithramycin was given. By that evening, his serum calcium had dropped to 14.3 mg/100 ml, and by the fourth day was down to 11.5 mg/100 ml. The patient's EKG pattern was now normal. Mithramycin was discontinued. The patient continued to receive palliative treatment for multiple myeloma.

In this patient, adequate hydration and saline infusion did not bring adequate diuresis. Despite repeated doses of furosemide, he showed symptoms of possible fluid overload. This may have been due to impaired renal function associated with multiple myeloma. In any case, a change in treatment was called for. Oral phosphates were not used in this patient because hypercalcemia of multiple myeloma does not respond well to them. Mithramycin was tried with good effect. This shows how the treatment of calcium imbalance must be personalized for each patient.

Calcium imbalance is not the most common electrolyte imbalance, but it can be a serious one. It requires immediate treatment — carefully planned for each patient.

Magnesium
THE FORGOTTEN ELECTROLYTE

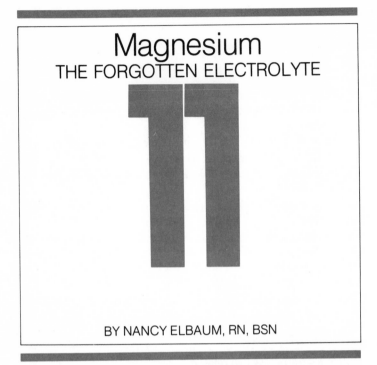

BY NANCY ELBAUM, RN, BSN

DO YOU USUALLY IGNORE MAGNESIUM when assessing a patient with fluid and electrolyte disorders? That's an understandable oversight since serum magnesium levels aren't usually included in routine tests for serum electrolytes. But magnesium imbalance can cause serious problems — from muscle weakness to life-threatening arrhythmias. And you should know about these.

The case of Mary Smith was typical. She was admitted with chronic diarrhea, weakness, and aversion to food. She had no history of similar episodes, weight loss, or a change in bowel habits. There was nothing to suggest food poisoning or toxic ingestion. Her blood tests showed a low calcium level, but treatment with calcium gluconate did not change her serum calcium level or her symptoms. We suspected magnesium deficit and ordered a serum determination, which showed 1.0 mEq/L (normal is 1.5 to 2.5 mEq/L).

Most magnesium-related disorders result from magnesium deficiency (hypomagnesemia). This deficiency does not usually follow inadequate dietary intake alone. Such deficiency only occurs when something impairs the absorption of magnesium, or excretion becomes too rapid. For example,

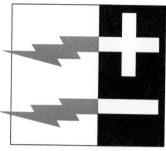

Profile on magnesium
Normal plasma value:
1.5 to 2.5 mEq/liter

MAGNESIUM FACTS
Magnesium helps cell
metabolism, activates many
enzyme systems, and influences
the metabolism of nucleic acids
and proteins. Magnesium also
affects skeletal muscle directly by
depressing acetylcholine release
at the synaptic junction; it
facilitates transportation of
sodium and potassium across
cell membranes (accounting for
the secondary hypokalemia that
occurs in hypomagnesemia); and
it influences intracellular calcium
levels through its effect on
parathyroid hormone secretion.

An adult body contains about
2,000 mEq of magnesium. Some
60% of it is in bone, about 1% in
extracellular fluid, and the rest in
muscle and other soft tissues. The
serum levels vary with the method
of determination, and may not
reflect total body stores of
magnesium.

A healthy person ingests about
25 mEq of magnesium daily,
mostly in meat, green vegetables,
whole grains, and nuts. About
10 mEq of magnesium are
absorbed daily through the small
bowel, and approximately the
same amount is excreted daily in
the urine. The rest is lost in the
stool. During hypomagnesemia,
however, the kidneys conserve
magnesium and excrete only
about 1 mEq per day.

hypomagnesemia is likely to show up in patients with these ailments:

Impaired absorption:
- malabsorption syndrome (e.g., nontropical sprue or steatorrhea) or chronic diarrhea
- bowel resection
- inherited intestinal defect in magnesium absorption.

Excessive renal excretion or fluid loss:
- prolonged parenteral fluid treatment without magnesium supplement
- alcoholism (diarrhea and inadequate diet may be contributing factors)
- hypercalcemic conditions, including hyperparathyroidism and malignancy
- diuretic therapy
- diabetic acidosis
- renal defect in magnesium reabsorption
- primary aldosteronism
- prolonged nasogastric suction.

Calcium and potassium related

When you find low calcium and low potassium levels, expect to see low magnesium levels too, for they frequently coexist. In fact, low calcium and potassium levels that do not respond to treatment with calcium and potassium replacement may point to hypomagnesemia. Remember that hypocalcemia due to magnesium deficiency disappears in about 4 days with appropriate magnesium replacement.

How to treat hypomagnesemia

Mild magnesium deficiency is usually treated with intramuscular injections of magnesium sulfate (8 to 16 mEq/L every 8 hours for 5 days), followed by a maintenance dose of 1 g (8 mEq) per day for as long as losses continue or serum magnesium depletion persists. A 50% solution is available in 2-ml vials for I.M. administration.

Magnesium sulfate (10%) is also available in a 10-ml (8 mEq) vial for addition to I.V. bottles, but intravenous use is usually reserved for severe or life-threatening situations.

Here are some things you should keep in mind when correcting magnesium deficiency:
- Watch for and avoid overcorrection to hypermagnesemia.

Some Magnesium Supplements		
PRODUCT	AMOUNT OF MAGNESIUM SUPPLIED	NURSING TIPS
Tablets Magora-Forte Mg-Plus Mg + C	30 mg 60 mg 20 mg	• Excessive doses may cause laxative effect; magnesium inhibits absorption of tetracycline
Solution Magnesium-Rougier◇◇	5 mg/ml	• Should be administered with caution
Parenteral Magnesium sulfate◇	10% solution (100 mg/ml) in 10, 20 ml ampules and 20 ml disposable units 25% solution (250 mg/ml) in 10 ml ampules 50% solution (500 mg/ml) in 2, 10, 20 ml ampules; 5, 10, 20 ml disposable units; and 30 ml vials	Magnesium sulfate is used as follows: • As a nutritional supplement in hyperalimentation • As an anticonvulsant, especially in pre-eclampsia or eclampsia • Administered I.V. diluted to a concentration of 20% or less • Administered deep I.M. 50% solution in adults; 20% in children • Use with caution in patients receiving diuretics, corticosteroids and CNS depressants

The symptoms of hypermagnesemia include flushing, sweating, and weak or absent deep tendon reflexes.

• Rate of infusion should not exceed 150 mg/minute. Rapid drip induces an uncomfortable feeling of heat.

• Do not give magnesium to patients with renal insufficiency. (If absolutely necessary, give magnesium with extreme caution.)

• During intravenous replacement of magnesium (especially if rapid), watch for respiratory depression or signs of heart block.

• Keep intravenous calcium gluconate on hand to reverse signs of magnesium intoxication.

• After replacement, re-test the patient frequently for magnesium depletion. If the patient continues to lose magnesium, he may become depleted again quickly.

Symptoms of magnesium imbalance

HYPOMAGNESEMIA

Central nervous system	Insomnia
Cardio-vascular	Leg and foot cramps; cardiac arrhythmias
Neuro-muscular	Muscle weakness, seizures, twitching, tremors, tetany

HYPERMAGNESEMIA

Central nervous system	Drowsiness, lethargy, diminished sensorium, coma
Cardio-vascular	Flushing, sweating, hypotension; slow weak pulse; bradycardia, heart block, cardiac arrest
Neuro-muscular	Diminished reflex or muscle weakness, flaccid paralysis
Respiratory	Respiratory depression

Hypermagnesemia: Often from self-medication

Expect to find magnesium excess in patients unable to excrete magnesium (as in chronic kidney failure) combined with excessive use of antacids (magnesium hydroxide), magnesium-containing cathartics such as Epsom salts, (magnesium sulfate), or milk of magnesia (magnesium hydroxide).

The symptoms of hypermagnesemia result from interference with neuromuscular transmission by excessive numbers of magnesium ions. These symptoms occur in a predictable pattern of progression, beginning with hypotension accompanied by flushing, a feeling of warmth, and sweating. These symptoms can appear at serum levels as low as 3 to 4 mEq/L. At serum levels of 10 mEq/L, deep tendon reflexes are weak or absent. At this level, the patient may also show flaccid paralysis; hypothermia; diminished cardiac function (slow, weak pulse); drowsiness; and other signs of CNS depression.

When you see any of these symptoms in a patient in whom you suspect hypermagnesemia, check the patellar reflex. If the reflex is diminished or absent, discontinue any magnesium the patient may be taking. At serum levels around 15 mEq/L, respiratory depression or paralysis may occur, so check the respiratory rate to be sure it is at least 16 per minute. When magnesium toxicity reaches 25 mEq/L, coma and cardiac arrest are likely to occur.

Chloride
CLUE TO ACIDITY

12

BY STANLEY GRISSINGER, BSc

EVEN THOUGH LABORATORY REPORTS routinely include serum chloride levels, nurses seldom worry about them — because changes in serum chloride *alone* rarely cause clinical problems. Mainly, they help identify acid-base imbalance; and they sometimes accompany other more significant deficits of potassium and sodium. Such clinical insignificance seems strange when you consider that chloride accounts for two-thirds of the total anions in the blood. And, chloride helps maintain water balance, osmotic pressure and the extracellular cation/anion balance. Nevertheless, it's true that chloride is most important clinically for its role in acid-base balance.

How does chloride tie in to acid-base balance?
Chloride competes with bicarbonate for combination with sodium ions. When chloride levels fall, the bicarbonate rises in compensation (because total anions must always equal total cations). In other words, extra bicarbonate ions are retained to balance the sodium ions. Thus, excessive loss of chloride-rich secretions such as gastric juice may cause alkalosis (hypochloremic metabolic alkalosis). Alkalosis causes hyperexcita-

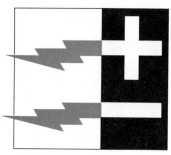

Profile on chloride
Normal plasma value:
95 to 109 mEq/liter

bility of the nervous system, especially of the peripheral nerves. So, to identify this condition, watch for hypertonicity of muscles, tetany, and depressed respirations.

On the other hand, excessive retention or ingestion of chloride ions releases extra bicarbonate ions from the kidney tubules, lowering the circulating base bicarbonate. This leads to *hyperchloremic metabolic acidosis,* a condition that depresses the central nervous system. To identify it, watch for stupor, deep rapid breathing, weakness and, in severe acidosis, coma (see Chapter 7).

Mr. Oliver's hypochloremic metabolic alkalosis resulted from excessive loss of chloride ions during 4 days of gastric suction. Sixty-four-year-old Seth Oliver developed paralytic ileus 3 days after abdominal surgery. Gastric suctioning removed more than 2 liters of secretions daily for 4 days. Despite replacement of gastrointestinal losses with sodium and potassium chloride, he became alkalotic on the seventh postoperative day. Laboratory values were: serum pH, 7.60; bicarbonate, 38 mEq/L; serum sodium, 140 mEq/L; serum potassium, 5.6 mEq/L; and serum chloride, 86 mEq/L. The doctor decided to correct Mr. Oliver's alkalosis with hydrochloric acid. After infusion of 2 liters of 0.1 normal (N) HCl through a central venous pressure (CVP) line at a rate of 1 liter daily, Mr. Oliver's chloride values became normal.

Loss of gastric secretions usually produces loss of potassium and sodium as well as chloride. Indeed, it is usually the loss or gain of these accompanying electrolytes that produces clinical problems. In Mr. Oliver's case, sodium and potassium losses were being replaced, and chloride deficit occurred alone.

Serum chloride values vary
Normal values for serum chloride range from 95 to 109 mEq/L. Several different assay methods can determine serum chloride levels, so individual labs may report slightly different normal values. Know what values your lab considers normal. Remember that blood samples should be processed promptly to prevent a chloride shift from plasma to red cells, causing falsely low values. Also, lab values for serum chloride may be falsely high or low if the patient is using certain drugs. Expect *high* chloride values if the patient's taking any of the following drugs: ammonium chloride; boric acid (toxicity); ion-

Some Commonly Used Chloride Supplements		
PRODUCT	AMOUNT OF CHLORIDE SUPPLIED	NURSING TIPS
Tablets Ammonium chloride	300 mg 500 mg 1 g (enteric coated)	• Large doses may cause metabolic acidosis due to hyperchloremia. May cause gastric irritation; absorption of enteric tablets is unpredictable; administer p.c.
Syrup Ammonium chloride	500 mg/5 ml	
Powder L-lysine monohydrochloride	Not available commercially	
Parenteral Arginine hydrochloride (R-Gene)	5% solution	• Rapid infusion may produce vomiting, irritation at infusion site, and acidosis (in patients with renal disease)
Hydrochloric acid	Not available commercially	• Pharmacy usually prepares a 0.1 normal HCl solution. Use extreme caution in transcribing the doctor's order. Errors have been reported in transcribing 100 mg HCl as 100 mEq of KCl!
Ammonium chloride○	0.6%/100 ml (11.2 mEq ammonium and chloride)	• Must be administered very slowly to avoid ammonium toxicity. Don't administer I.M. or S.C.

exchange resins cholestyramine (Questran); oxyphenbutazone (Tandearil); phenylbutazone (Butazolidin); and excess intravenous sodium chloride.

Also expect *high* chloride values in patients with dehydration when chloride ions become concentrated in decreased volume. Hyperchloremia may also occur: in head injury (which causes neurogenic hyperventilation); in primary hyperparathyroidism (in which the kidneys waste phosphates, and chloride levels rise); in metabolic acidosis (because excreted bicarbonate ions are replaced by chloride ions); and finally, in respiratory alkalosis (low carbonic acid is usually due to hyperventilation, which blows off carbon dioxide). The only treatment for hyperchloremia is removal of the underlying disease or the pharmacologic stimulus.

Expect *low* chloride values if the patient is taking: bicarbonate; ethacrynic acid (Edecrin); furosemide (Lasix); thiazide diuretics; or 5% dextrose in water for prolonged I.V. use (dilutional effect).

Trace elements

More than fifty elements occur in minute quantities in human tissues. These so-called trace elements influence many physiologic processes including enzyme function and protein and nucleic acid synthesis.

So far, only a handful of trace elements are known to cause clinical deficiency states:

• *Cobalt* is an essential component of vitamin B_{12}. Its deficiency can cause pernicious anemia.

• *Copper* deficiency has been implicated in an anemia that mimics iron-deficiency anemia. Copper-free diets have led to leukopenia and neutropenia.

• *Iodine* is essential for thyroid function. Iodine deficiency leads to hypothyroidism.

• *Zinc* appears to be necessary for wound healing and enzyme activity. In at least one patient on long-term hyperalimentation, zinc deficiency was associated with acrodermatitis enteropathica, a syndrome of diarrhea, mental depression, oral lesions, and alopecia.

• *Manganese* seems essential for skeletal growth and calcium and phosphorous metabolism.

Normal diets and most dietary supplements and vitamins with minerals easily provide the necessary trace elements. But hyperalimentation fluids do not. So, consider the need for trace element supplements for patients who must receive hyperalimentation for three weeks or more. Solutions containing trace elements must be compounded by the pharmacy since none are available commercially.

Usually, when chloride levels are low, so are potassium and sodium levels. The clinical signs are those you'd expect with potassium and sodium depletion. Expect low serum chloride levels in patients with: *hyperhidrosis* (excess chloride loss in perspiration); *gastrointestinal* disease (if suction or vomiting is prolonged); *acidosis* (in diabetic ketosis, ketonic anions replace chloride in the serum); *congestive heart failure* or *edema* (leads to extracellular fluid excess); *urinary losses* (chronic renal failure); *low-salt diet*; or *metabolic alkalosis*.

Hypochloremia can be corrected by chloride replacement. But that usually is not done; rather, treatment focuses on the underlying disease. When necessary, the following can supply chloride and correct alkalosis: ammonium chloride, L-lysine monohydrochloride, and arginine hydrochloride (which is presently in favor). If arginine is unavailable, intravenous solutions containing 100 mEq of hydrogen and 100 mEq of chloride per liter (0.1 N HCl in 5% dextrose) can be specially prepared by the hospital pharmacy. This solution is usually administered slowly through a central venous line.

Looking back to Mr. Oliver's case, we see that chloride could also have been replaced with L-lysine monohydrochloride, ammonium chloride, or arginine hydrochloride instead of hydrochloric acid. But, L-lysine must be given orally and this patient was not permitted anything by mouth. Ammonium chloride given intravenously can dangerously elevate serum ammonia levels. Arginine wasn't available, so hydrochloric acid was used and did reverse systemic alkalosis.

How to calculate the amount of chloride replacement? Use the following formula:

Cl deficit = (0.2) x (Wt. in kg) x (102 − observed Cl value)

Since Mr. Oliver weighed 67 kg and his chloride level was 86 mEq/L, he needed 214 milliequivalents of chloride:

(0.2) x (67 kg) x (102 − 86 mEq/L) = 214 mEq Cl

Since the hydrochloric acid solution contains (100 mEq/L), this represents 2.14 liters. He received 2 liters of this solution over 48 hours and did well.

SKILLCHECK 3

1. Sally Johnson is a 34-year-old brittle diabetic, admitted in diabetic ketoacidosis. Upon admission, her serum blood sugar was 640 mg per 100 ml. Her pH was 7.2; HCO_3^- 7 mEq; and her serum potassium, 6.2 mEq/L. Her initial treatment included I.V. glucose and regular insulin. What do you expect will happen to her serum potassium levels?

2. How can certain diuretics (mercurials, ethacrynic acid, and furosemide) cause alkalosis?

3. Mr. Puff, a 53-year-old tourist, was found mugged near the train station. On admission to the ED, he was unconscious and found to be in respiratory acidosis. He was intubated and placed on a volume respirator.

He was admitted to ICU with a severe concussion. Four hours later, while doing a neurological assessment, his nurse noticed muscle twitching and some widening of the Q-T interval on the monitor. She notified the doctor, who ordered *stat* electrolytes and arterial blood gases.

The results showed marked respiratory alkalosis. Electrolytes showed hypocalcemia, although they had been normal when drawn in the ED earlier. His symptoms of tetany were more pronounced and he was starting to seizure. So the doctor ordered an injection of 1 g of 10% calcium gluconate I.V.

His seizures stopped almost immediately after the injection of calcium. He remained stable for about 30 minutes, but then his nurse noticed atrial tachycardia with 2:1 block. By this time, Mr. Puff's wife had finally been reached by phone, and had told the doctor that her husband had chronic obstructive pulmonary disease, and was on digitalis. What caused this patient's hypocalcemia and arrhythmia? How could they have been prevented?

4. Mr. Lloyd, a 79-year-old retired bricklayer, was hospitalized with a fever of 104° F. (40.0° C.). His family tells you he's been quite sick for the past 5 days and hasn't been eating or drinking well. His skin feels hot and dry. His initial electrolytes are: Na, 154 mEq/L; K, 4 mEq/L; CO_2, 24; Cl, 96 mEq/L. How would you expect to treat his hypernatremia?

5. Ida Henry, a 46-year-old woman, had been admitted to the hospital for evaluation of severe back pain and a possible vertebral fracture at the level of T_{10}-T_{12}. She had a left radical mastectomy 2 years ago and may have metastasis to the bone. What would you expect her serum calcium to be? What treatment would you anticipate?

(Answers on page 198)

MANAGING SPECIAL PATIENTS

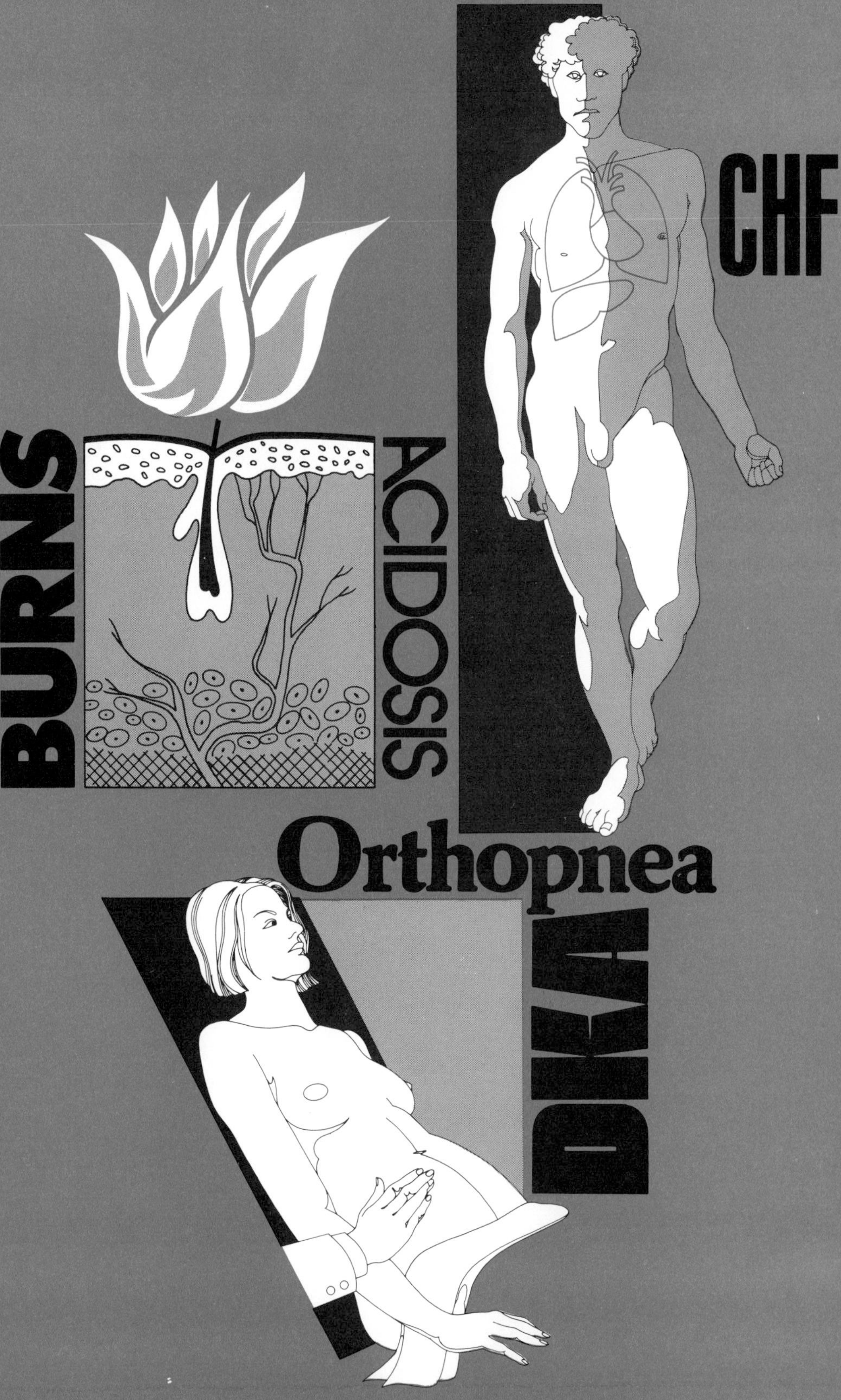

CHF

BURNS

ACIDOSIS

Orthopnea

DKA

Renal Failure
IMBALANCES INEVITABLE

13

BY JUNE L. STARK, RN

DO YOU KNOW HOW to recognize the various stages of renal failure? How to correlate changes in renal status with fluids, diet, and medications? Such skills are necessary if you are to help the patient in renal failure to regain some of his compromised function.

Consider the case of Jane Newton. Ms. Newton, a 31-year-old teacher, with a history of post-streptococcal glomerulonephritis, was hospitalized with an E-Coli urinary tract infection. Before this admission, her renal function tests showed a serum creatinine of 3. She had no complaints except for "occasional accumulation of fluid in her ankles." When this happened, she would restrict her salt intake. Her complaints on admission were: decreasing urinary output; dark urine; burning; urgency and frequency; plus rapid weight gain (5 pounds over 2 days). At admission, she weighed 125 lbs and had ankle edema, which was pitting, and her serum creatinine was up to 6. Her blood pressure was slightly elevated, and she had a temperature of 101° F. (38.3° C.). The doctor ordered a 10-day treatment with antibiotics. A 24-hour urine collection was started for creatinine clearance to accurately measure the glomerular filtration rate (GFR) and proteins in order to assess her renal status and compare it to her previous admission.

Urinalysis showed gross hematuria, proteinuria, 4+ WBC, WBC casts (both, signs of infection) and bacteria. The nurse examined the urine for color, concentration, and odor. She measured the specific gravity at 1.020 (within upper normal limits). The pH was 6.5, and the sugar and acetone were negative. Even though her serum creatinine had risen, Ms. Newton still had a normal serum K+ and Na+, despite her decreased urine output. So, she still had the capacity to concentrate urine. She was assessed as having moderate renal insufficiency.

An intake and output sheet was started, and initially Ms. Newton was allowed to drink an amount which equaled urine output plus 750 ml. The next day, her 24-hour urine showed: 4 g protein and a decreased creatinine clearance. After 7 days of antibiotics, her urine culture was negative; her urine output was increasing; and her serum creatinine was falling. Fluid restriction was removed, and she was discharged on a 2 g per day sodium and high-protein diet. She was taught how to record her daily body weight; estimate her urine output; and report signs and symptoms immediately.

Each stage of renal failure has its own characteristic signs and symptoms. You need to know what these symptoms are, how severe a failure they represent, and how to devise a care plan accordingly. Do not assume that all renal failure patients require fluid and dietary restrictions. Some patients with renal failure present with polyuria, salt-wasting, and proteinuria. They need forced fluids plus a high-sodium and high-protein diet.

Only after thoroughly assessing renal status, can you make sound judgments on medication dosage, diet, and fluid administration.

What happens in renal disease?

Nephrons are uniquely adaptable to some loss of their population. The remaining healthy nephrons then work at supernormal capacity to handle a higher solute and water load. Indeed, up to 75% of total nephrons can be lost before signs of end-stage renal disease become evident. This ability of the nephron to compensate for a slowly progressing disease results in the varying degrees of renal insufficiency that we see in our patients. The signs and symptoms of chronic renal disease vary according to which part of the nephron is damaged — the glomerulus or the tubules.

Glomerular disease

The most common glomerular disease is glomerulonephritis. This disease has an immunologic basis and causes changes in the glomerular membrane and/or cellular structure. In a diseased state, the glomerulus loses its ability to be semipermeable. Protein and red blood cells then filter through the glomerular capillary walls into the urine. Proteinuria and hematuria develop.

In early glomerulonephritis, the GFR can be normal or moderately depressed. As the disease progresses, and a large number of glomeruli are involved, the urine output can decrease (oliguria — less than 600 ml/24 hours).

So let's review: With glomerular disease, expect to see a normal-to-decreasing urine output, proteinuria which may exceed 2 to 4 grams, and hematuria. In end-stage glomerulonephritis, the damage will eventually involve the tubules.

Tubular disease

The most common chronic disease affecting the tubules is interstitial nephritis. In patients with this disease, the tubular cells are damaged and are unable to selectively reabsorb and excrete the components needed for homeostasis. Since the tubular cells cannot concentrate the urine, the filtrate moves along the tubule and is excreted essentially unchanged. In patients with this disease (if there is no obstruction), expect to see decreased GFR, polyuria, acid-base imbalance and possibly salt-wasting syndrome.

As the total number of nephrons (glomeruli and tubules) diminishes, the kidney gradually loses its ability to excrete waste products, and to preserve homeostasis. Eventually, end-stage renal disease evolves, with azotemia, possibly progressing to uremia, elevated serum creatinine levels, and oliguria or anuria.

Clues to assessment

When you care for a patient you suspect has renal disease, always begin with a history and physical assessment. Ask yourself:
- Has the patient been told he has renal disease in the past?

Filtering the flow

In the healthy kidney, the glomerulus, a capillary bed, filters about 120 ml of plasma a minute through its semipermeable membrane. The "glomerular filtrate" or "ultrafiltrate" that results forms the main component of urine. The rate of formation, or glomerular filtration rate (GFR), helps measure the degree of renal function.

These factors decrease the GFR and the formation of urine:
- dehydration or decreased extracellular fluid volume
- hypotension
- decreased cardiac output
- hyponatremia
- renal disease: obstruction and glomerular disease

These factors increase the GFR and the formation of urine:
- overhydration or increased extracellular fluid volume
- hypertension
- increased cardiac output
- hypernatremia
- renal disease: tubular-medullary disease.

Kidneys — the regulating pair

As you know, the kidneys rid the body of waste, regulate the chemical makeup and pressure of the blood, and maintain a proper balance of fluid and electrolytes. One kidney comprises approximately one million nephrons, the structural and functional unit of the organ. The microscopic nephron is made up of two parts, the glomerulus and the tubules. The tubules are further divided into segments: proximal, loop of Henle, and distal and collecting ducts. Each segment plays a role in the retention and excretion of water, electrolytes, and waste products.

The glomerulus, a capillary bed, filters the blood to produce a filtrate. Any unfiltered plasma returns to the systemic blood supply, while the filtrate flows along the length of the tubules. The tubular cells reabsorb the necessary water, nutrients, and electrolytes and excrete the metabolic waste products (urea and creatinine), hydrogen ions, and other excesses.

Each day 180 liters of plasma is formed into filtrate: One liter is excreted as urine and the remaining 179 liters are reabsorbed by the tubules. This relationship of blood flow to the kidney, normal glumerular and tubular function, antidiuretic hormone, and the renin-aldosterone system determines the fluid, sodium, and potassium balance in the body and the composition of the urine.

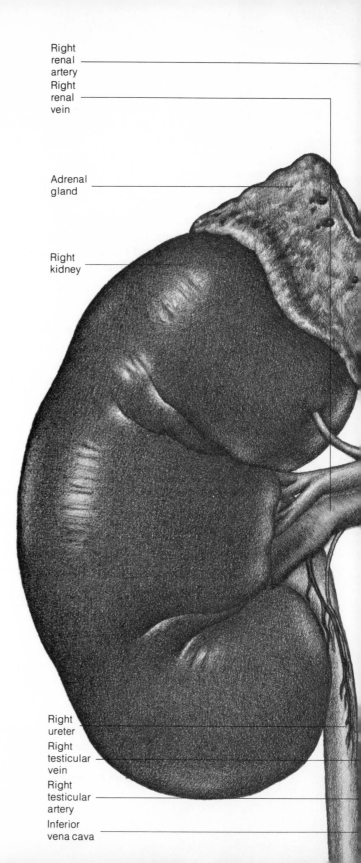

Right renal artery

Right renal vein

Adrenal gland

Right kidney

Right ureter

Right testicular vein

Right testicular artery

Inferior vena cava

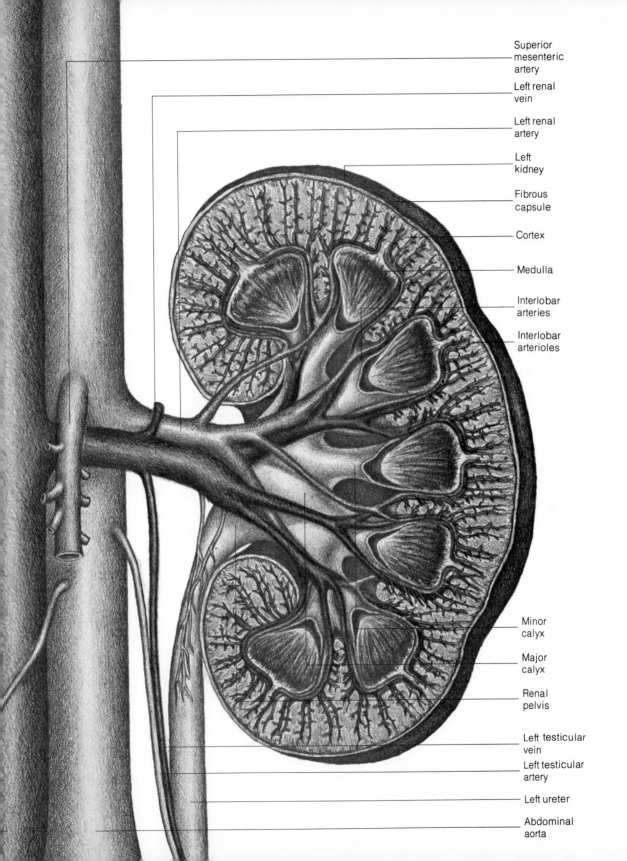

Superior
mesenteric
artery

Left renal
vein

Left renal
artery

Left
kidney

Fibrous
capsule

Cortex

Medulla

Interlobar
arteries

Interlobar
arterioles

Minor
calyx

Major
calyx

Renal
pelvis

Left testicular
vein

Left testicular
artery

Left ureter

Abdominal
aorta

Four stages of renal deterioration

Here's a handy set of definitions to help you assess your patient's renal function.

DIMINISHED RENAL RESERVE — Although kidney function as a whole is mildly reduced, the excretory and regulatory functions sufficiently maintain a normal internal environment.

RENAL INSUFFICIENCY — Some evidences of impaired capacity may appear in the form of mild azotemia, slightly impaired concentrating ability, and anemia. However, these abnormalities are minimal until dehydration, infection, heart failure and so on put stress on the kidney.

RENAL FAILURE — Kidney function has deteriorated to the point of chronic and persistent abnormalities in the internal environment.

UREMIC SYNDROME — Many clinical signs and symptoms may appear in the patient with renal failure.

- If so, what are his symptoms?
- Is there a family history of kidney disease?
- Is there a history of diabetes or high blood pressure?
- Has he noticed a variation in frequency or quantity of urination?
- What does his urine look like?
- Does he complain of nocturia; excessive thirst; unusual fatigue; weight change; edema; or burning, urgency, or frequency of urination?
- Why did he come to the hospital?

Recognizing sudden changes in the patient's condition is very important. In most renal disease, kidney function remains fairly consistent unless the disease process is temporarily exacerbated by other problems such as congestive heart failure, dehydration, and infection. Then, you may notice a sudden rise in serum creatinine and urea nitrogen, plus a sharp decrease in urine output associated with weight gain.

Nursing care of patients with renal disease focuses on three essential goals: managing fluids, keeping electrolytes balanced, and regulating the dosage of medication.

Managing fluids

Daily body weights and 24-hour totals of intake and output (I and O) are mandatory. Your record of intake and output should include all possible sources of intake (I.V., oral, and irrigation) and all output (nasogastric tube, wound drainage). By maintaining a "running cumulative balance" (total the sheet every hour) you can see the patient's fluid status at all times. If hourly totals are impossible, total the amounts at least every 8 hours, and record a "total cumulative balance" at the end of 24 hours.

First, add up the I and O volume separately, then take two other things into consideration: *insensible loss* and *catabolic rate*. The insensible loss is the amount of water and electrolytes excreted daily via the skin, lungs, and bowels. An average estimate of this loss is 750 ml per day. The catabolic rate is assessed as the fluid gained by the metabolism of the carbohydrates obtained in dietary intake. This amount of fluid is approximately 350 ml. These amounts vary: insensible loss can be *increased* by fever and diaphoresis; catabolic rate can be *increased* by burns, massive trauma, infection, and most debilitating conditions. You must consider these variations to accurately measure the body's fluid status.

The last step is to incorporate all these values into your final balance. If the patient's:

• *fluid intake exceeds* the output, he is in a *positive balance* and *volume expansion* can result

• *fluid output exceeds* the intake, he is in a *negative* balance and *volume contraction* can result.

This is your estimate of *total body fluid balance* (TBFB). Check the patient's daily weight against the total body fluid balance (TBFB). An excess of 500 ml of fluid equals 1 lb of body weight. Rapid variations in weight closely reflect changes in fluid volume. Thus, the fluid and electrolyte regimen, diet, and the diuretic treatment depend daily on the total body fluid balance, weight, body temperature, and laboratory data.

The anuric patient will require a slightly different method since his kidneys cannot excrete sodium, water, and potassium. He may receive fluid totaling his insensible loss (750 ml) minus some of the water gained by ingestion of food (catabolic rate). But in complicated cases, the patient would receive less — a total of approximately 600 ml per day. Always incorporate the catabolic rate into the intake column since it can reveal volume excess (which is hazardous to the patient prone to edema and congestive heart failure).

Maintaining adequate hydration helps sustain renal function and improve the patient's overall condition. Adequate hydration prevents a drop in extracellular fluid volume (ECFV) and a drop in blood pressure which can further compromise the existing renal disease; excess ECFV can produce peripheral edema and, eventually, congestive heart failure.

Electrolyte and dietary management

Generally, the patient with renal disease needs some restriction of protein, sodium, and potassium. In kidney disease, the end-product of protein metabolism tends to accumulate. So, dietary limitation of protein is usually logical. Extreme restriction would be to 20 g/protein a day; liberal, to 60 g/day. Each diet should contain protein high in nutritive value (that is the essential amino acids, and calories). To determine which is the best diet, refer to the results of the 24-hour urine collection for protein. Is the patient losing large amounts of protein in his urine? If so, his diet will need to replace lost protein.

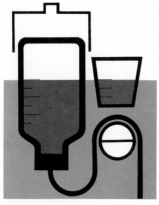

What to know
Here's a checklist to help you obtain the information you need to devise your patient's care plan.
1. Obtain laboratory results:
    Serum electrolytes: check for imbalances, depletion, or excess
    Urine electrolytes: check for wasting of salt or potassium
    Urinalysis: look for tubular casts, protein, RBCs, and WBCs
    Urine specific gravity: rule out dehydration and inability to concentrate urine
    Urine osmolality, pH, sugar, and acetone
    Inspect urine for color, odor, concentration, and sediment
    Collect urine over 24 hours for protein and creatinine clearance
2. Physical assessment:
    Obtain patient's weight
    Check skin turgor and mucous membranes
    Record any signs of edema
    Check pain over kidney to rule out infection
    Check for pain, urgency, and burning upon urination
3. Note any evidence of heart or liver disease as well as any other complications that might affect treatment
4. Measure all drainage such as vomiting, diarrhea, draining wounds, fistulas, and GI suction, and send specimen to lab for electrolyte content.

The other waste product that accumulates in renal failure is creatinine. Creatinine is the product of muscle activity, and its blood levels will not be changed by diet or most conservative treatment methods.

Follow essentially the same steps for determining sodium and potassium intake. Check the serum and urine levels. If the kidneys cannot excrete the electrolytes, then limit their dietary intake. If large amounts are lost in the urine, replace the deficiency. Then consider two situations that demand restriction. If the patient has hypertension or edema, strict sodium restriction is necessary. If he has an increased catabolic rate and tissue destruction, intracellular *potassium* will enter the serum, and strict potassium restriction will be necessary.

In chronic renal disease, the remaining nephrons may adjust to the increased potassium load. But watch for hyperkalemia, especially during acute exacerbations of renal disease. Other than diet, there's one conservative way to remove excess serum potassium: sodium polystyrene sulfonate (Kayexalate), a cation-exchange resin. The usual dosage is 50 to 100 g mixed with 50 to 100 ml of sorbitol and water, given by mouth or enema. This removes potassium from the body by a process in which 1 mEq of Na^+ is exchanged for 1 mEq of K^+, while the sorbitol causes an osmotic diarrhea. This method can remove as much potassium as 0.5 to 1 mEq/L per treatment. However, this method replaces sodium for the potassium it removes, so be alert for signs of hypernatremia.

When dialysis?
The patient with renal failure needs some form of dialysis when he develops uremic symptoms, uncontrollable hyperkalemia, congestive heart failure, or uncontrollable acidosis.

Monitor medications
Drugs get excreted by the kidneys. So, dosage becomes a problem when a needed drug is directly excreted by the kidneys but renal function is inadequate. You must carefully adjust drug dosage or time intervals to avoid toxic accumulation in the body.

The doctor will initially calculate the drug dosage according to GFR and creatinine clearance. Your duty is to question this dosage whenever the patient shows a sudden rise in serum creatinine or any other signs of deteriorating renal function.

Congestive Heart Failure
FLUID PROBLEMS CRITICAL

14

BY BARBARA BONAVENTURA, RN, BSN

DO YOU FEEL COMPLETELY competent when you know your next patient has acute congestive heart failure (CHF)? As you await his arrival, you know he's likely to have a multitude of problems. Not the least of these will be fluid and electrolyte imbalance. Such imbalances are inevitable and prominent in congestive heart failure. Why inevitable? Because fluid and electrolyte disturbances stem from the disease itself and from its treatment.

How CHF produces fluid imbalance
Congestive heart failure produces fluid imbalance via several interlocking mechanisms. For example, edema develops because:

• decreased renal blood flow increases secretion of aldosterone (as much as triple the normal amount) causing sodium and water retention.

• liver congestion, a result of increased venous blood volume, may aggravate edema by preventing inactivation of aldosterone and ADH (which are normally inactivated by the liver).

• excessive venous blood volume increases hydrostatic

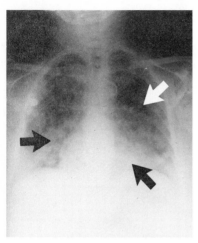

Now you see them
You can diagnose and evaluate the severity of congestive heart failure and pulmonary edema with chest X-rays like the one above. Notice the presence of hilar congestion and the prominence of pulmonary vascular markings. These "butterfly or bat-wing configurations," as they are sometimes called, indicate congestion. Notice, too, how enlarged the patient's heart has become.

pressure and, so, shifts fluid from the intravascular to the interstitial compartment.

At the same time, electrolyte imbalances develop because:
• excessive aldosterone secretion promotes potassium excretion and leads to potassium deficit.

• diuretics also waste potassium and lead to its deficit.

• mercurial and thiazide diuretics cause selective excretion of more chloride ions than sodium ions; chloride loss brings compensatory increase in bicarbonate ions, hence metabolic alkalosis.

• pulmonary congestion interferes with the elimination of carbon dioxide from the lungs and leads to respiratory acidosis.

• extensive use of diuretics plus severely restricted sodium intake lead to sodium deficit.

Mr. Tarleton's history shows fluid and electrolyte problems so characteristic in congestive heart failure.

Mr. Tarleton, a 65-year-old retired machinist, was hospitalized with irregular heartbeat. He'd recently developed increasingly frequent dyspnea upon climbing stairs and occasionally suffered paroxysmal nocturnal dyspnea. He had extreme fatigue, orthopnea that required him to sleep on two pillows, and nocturia that awakened him at least twice each night. Physical examination revealed distended neck veins, bibasilar rales, and an irregular tachycardia. (EKG findings were uncontrolled atrial fibrillation with frequent premature ventricular contractions of more than 8 per minute.) He had no visible edema.

Mr. Tarleton was admitted to the coronary care unit for control of his congestive heart failure and associated pulmonary edema. A lidocaine bolus (50 mg) was given first, followed by lidocaine drip for his ventricular irritability. His pulmonary artery mean pressure was 35, which is extremely high (normal, 15). To reduce his pulmonary congestion and the heart rate, treatment began with furosemide (Lasix) 120 mg I.V. and digoxin (Lanoxin) 0.25 mg I.V. (times 3). An I.V. of 500 ml of 5% dextrose in water (to run slowly) was started as an open line for medications. Lab studies showed serum sodium, 130; potassium, 4.0; and some renal impairment. Blood urea nitrogen was 40; creatinine, 2.5.

Within 24 hours, Mr. Tarleton's pulmonary pressure fell to 23 and bibasilar rales had diminished. (A mean pulmonary pressure of 23 is normally considered high, but in this case it probably was at a tolerable level.) During this time, Mr. Tarleton was restricted to bedrest in semi-Fowler's position. His respiratory distress had disappeared, and lab studies showed improved renal function. Sodium restriction was ordered (to 2 g sodium/day) but fluid restriction was not. Three days after admission, his serum sodium levels were essentially unchanged. Supplementary potassium (20 mEq/L in 5% dextrose and water) was administered through the I.V., and serum levels remained between 3.9 to 4.5. He was continued on daily oral doses of digoxin, 0.25 mg and furosemide, 40 mg. His pulse stabilized between 90 and 100 but continued to be somewhat irregular.

Five days after admission, Mr. Tarleton began gradually to increase his physical activity and was transferred to a medical unit for continued treatment. Now an important nursing objective was educating Mr. Tarleton about his disease and therapy. He received diet instructions on sodium restriction and a list of foods to avoid. His activity was strictly regulated to avoid activity that would precipitate dyspnea. At this time, he was able to take charge of his personal care and tolerate moderate exercise without dyspnea or pain.

At discharge (after 12 days), Mr. Tarleton knew the dosage, frequency of administration, and side effects of his medications; he knew how to restrict his sodium and supplement his potassium; and he knew his activity limitations. At discharge, he had no edema, no bibasilar rales, and no neck vein distention. His pulse continued to be irregular at a rate of 90 to 100. He was to return to his doctor for follow-up.

As you know, congestive heart failure is not an isolated event but a chain of deficits that lead to a complex response by all the body systems. Because of this, your nursing observations and care are crucial and can profoundly affect the outcome of treatment. Your observations should begin at admission with baseline assessment of the patient's physical and mental status. Of course, this assessment should always include the patient's weight and vital signs, temperature, pulse, respiration, and blood pressure. Look at the patient. Observe his appearance and behavior and take a thorough nursing history. Obviously, you don't need to complete all of his history at admission, especially if the patient is in great distress when admitted. However, noting his physical appearance,

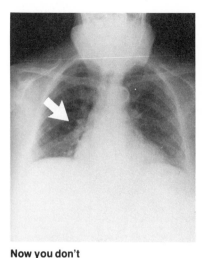

Now you don't
The X-ray above was taken of the same patient after four days of treatment for congestive failure and pulmonary edema. This patient was treated with diuretics, digoxin, and bedrest, which reduced the pulmonary congestion as you can see by the decrease in vascular markings. The size of the patient's heart was also reduced as the congestion was relieved, and cardiac output improved.

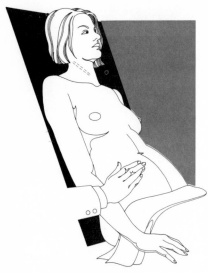

A pressing concern
In patients with right-sided heart
failure you can detect venous
congestion early by evaluating
the hepato-jugular reflex. Place
the patient in a semi-Fowler's
position so that she is elevated
enough for the blood column of
her jugular vein to be visible
above the clavicle.
    Have the patient relax and
breathe normally. Now place your
hand on her abdomen. As you
press firmly toward the right upper
quadrant and under the costal
margin, watch the blood column
of her jugular vein. If she has
venous congestion, the pressure
you apply will displace a small
amount of blood from the liver and
cause her jugular vein to distend
about 1 to 2 cm.

mental state, and vital signs is mandatory to provide a baseline
for measuring effects of treatment.

Symptoms may vary
Does right-sided or left-sided failure predominate initially?
The patient's symptoms may vary accordingly. In left-sided
failure, decreased cardiac output produces cyanosis, fatigue
and disorientation. Blood backs up in the pulmonary circulatory system. Left-sided failure is the kind most likely to occur
after myocardial infarction. Its symptoms reflect: increased
congestion and pressure within the pulmonary system and
decreased blood flow to all tissues and organs. In patients with
left-sided failure, expect to see dyspnea on exertion or at rest,
tachypnea, orthopnea, paroxysmal nocturnal dyspnea, cough,
pulmonary rales (which may be audible *without* a stethoscope), fatigue, mental confusion, sodium and water retention,
and decreased tolerance to physical activity.

   Right-sided failure may follow left-sided failure because the
right side must pump against the increased resistance in the
pulmonary system that results from left-sided failure. Right-
sided failure may also follow: obstructive pulmonary disease,
pulmonary embolism, emphysema, asthma, and chronic
bronchitis. When right-sided failure results from lung disease,
it's called cor pulmonale.

   Patients with right-sided failure characteristically develop
dependent edema, coolness of the extremities, hepatomegaly,
aching abdominal pain, ascites, neck vein distention, and increased venous pressure. They usually show a positive hepa-
tojugular reflex. (If you apply pressure to the patient's abdomen above the liver, the jugular vein becomes distended.)

Three goals of treatment
Treatment of congestive heart failure aims to:
1. Eliminate the cause whenever possible (as in surgical correction of incompetent or stenosed valves).
2. Establish cardiac output adequate for metabolic needs by:
— increasing the force of myocardial contraction with digitalis and by
— reducing the demand on cardiac output by reducing physical activity; and
3. Correct fluid congestion and electrolyte imbalances by:
reducing circulatory blood volume with diuretics; reducing

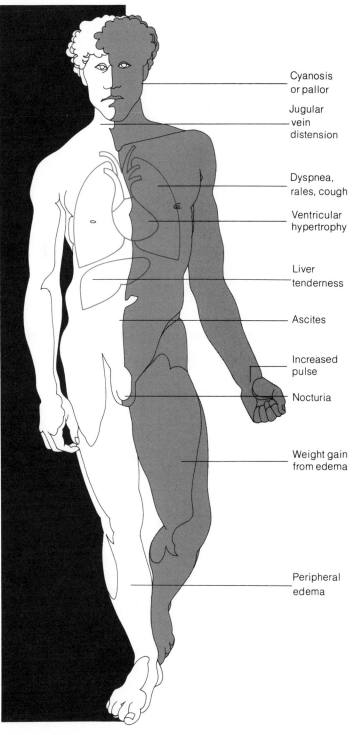

Cyanosis or pallor

Jugular vein distension

Dyspnea, rales, cough

Ventricular hypertrophy

Liver tenderness

Ascites

Increased pulse

Nocturia

Weight gain from edema

Peripheral edema

Two pumps in one

Consider the heart as two pumps, one on the right and one on the left. Each side depends on the other for its own efficiency since the failure of one pump will eventually affect the other. If you understand the symptoms associated with right- and left-sided heart failure, as shown here, you will sharpen your assessment skills and be more helpful to your patient.

SYMPTOMS OF HEART FAILURE
Right side
Jugular vein distension
Liver tenderness
Ascites
Nocturia
Peripheral edema
Left side
Cyanosis or pallor
Dyspnea, rales, cough
Ventricular hypertrophy
Increased pulse
Weight gain from edema

A big heart

Any pathological process (such as mitral insufficiency, atrial or ventricular septal defects, or tricuspid insufficiency) can produce an overload of blood in the ventricles. This stretches or strains the myocardial fibers in the ventricles, resulting in hypertrophy. You can see these hypertrophic changes on an EKG in leads oriented to the specific ventricle involved.

You can see left ventricular hypertrophy (LVH) in leads oriented to the left ventricle, V4, V5, and V6, (shown on this page). Notice a tall R wave in these leads, taller than the S wave; S-T segment depression; and T wave changes. The QRS duration is usually prolonged but not longer than 0.12 seconds. These changes represent delay and alteration of conduction from the increased muscle mass.

You can see right ventricular hypertrophy (RVH) in leads oriented to the right ventricle, AVR, V2, and V3 (page 131). Notice tall R waves, taller than the S wave; S-T segment depression; and T wave inversion. Leads V1 and AVF also show these changes.

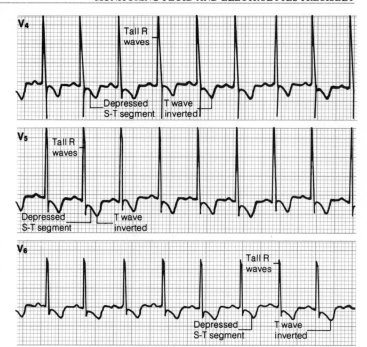

sodium concentration with diuretics and dietary restriction; and by maintaining normal serum potassium levels with potassium supplements, and potassium-sparing diuretics in combination with thiazides.

Correcting fluid congestion

Of course, what you do about fluids in a particular patient depends on his clinical status. He's likely to need therapy and careful monitoring to avoid fluid overload if he's already edematous. For this reason, strict intake and output records are always mandatory in the hospitalized patient with congestive heart failure.

If he can tolerate oral food and fluids, fluid restriction is generally unnecessary — mainly because of the efficiency of diuretics. Of course, when diuretics cannot reduce fluid congestion, fluid restriction is the only recourse. Keep in mind that, whether or not fluid intake is restricted, you must constantly watch every patient with congestive heart failure for signs of circulatory overload (increased CVP, moist rales, edema, and acute weight gain). Daily monitoring of the patient's body weight, venous pressure, strict intake and out-

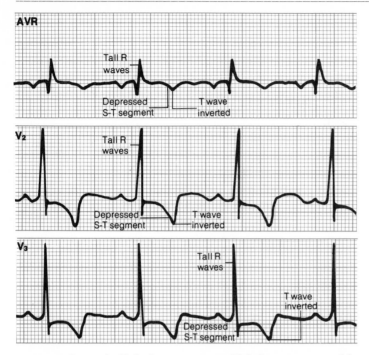

AVR

Tall R waves

Depressed S-T segment   T wave inverted

V₂

Tall R waves

Depressed S-T segment   T wave inverted

V₃

Tall R waves

T wave inverted

Depressed S-T segment

put records, and clinical symptoms will help you assess his fluid status correctly.

When fluid restriction is necessary, managing the patient can be difficult indeed. Carefully explain to him how much fluid he can have daily (often a total of only 1500 ml/day that includes both intravenous and oral intake) and why not more. Allow him to decide how he will distribute his small oral allowance during the day. This small chance to control his environment may help him overcome any resistance he may feel to this difficult restriction. If he complains of thirst, you can help by offering good mouth care — mouthwash or glycerine swabs — at least three times a day.

Heart failure may become refractory — not respond to treatment with diuretics or sodium restriction. That'll require restriction of fluid intake as low as 500 ml/day or rarely, paracentesis or thoracentesis. Paracentesis (removal of fluid from peritoneal cavity) will be needed if severe ascites interferes with respiratory function by compressing the diaphragm. Thoracentesis (removal of fluid from the pleural cavity) will be needed if fluid accumulation within the pleural cavity compromises respiratory function.

Correcting electrolytes

Sodium and potassium are the two electrolytes most affected by CHF and its treatment. The disease itself increases retention of sodium; the treatment aims to decrease extracellular sodium content and incidentally, wastes potassium. Nevertheless, sodium restriction is not always necessary because potent diuretics aid its excretion along with water. So, depending on individual response to diuretics, sodium restriction will vary. A sodium-restricted diet may allow as little as 200 to 600 mg/daily (as compared to the normal 3 g daily).

If your patient needs sodium restriction, you can help him by giving specific diet instructions. Include a resource list of high-sodium foods and show him how to recognize less obvious forms of sodium described on labels. Point out the many words that indicate sodium (salt and any words containing "sodium" or "monosodium glutamate"). Point out that low-sodium food can be made more palatable with salt substitutes. But warn the patient with heart failure against using substitutes containing potassium if he has any renal dysfunction. Educate the patient to the reasons for this difficult diet. Help him understand the consequences of noncompliance — increased breathing discomfort and swollen legs.

Hyponatremia is common in CHF. It may result from a dilutional effect (edema), from excessive sodium restriction, and any acute fluid loss (phlebotomy, diaphoresis, diarrhea, or centesis). So, if a sodium-restricted patient develops weakness, nausea and vomiting, or lethargy, check his serum sodium level for deficit. A slight increase in dietary sodium or an adjustment in diuretic dosage may be needed.

Remember to watch sodium-restricted patients more carefully for sodium deficit during hot weather. Heavy perspiring may call for more sodium than diet provides. Again, if hyponatremia appears, sodium allowance may need to be increased. Symptoms of severe sodium depletion include abdominal cramps, diarrhea, convulsions and apprehension.

Also, watch *potassium* levels carefully. During potent diuretic therapy, the body loses large amounts of potassium. If potassium supplements are not provided, the patient can develop serious deficit. Signs of digoxin toxicity are aversion to food, nausea and vomiting, diarrhea, confusion, and cardiac arrhythmias (severe bradycardia, ectopic ventricular beats), and atrial tachyarrhythmias with block.

Respiratory Failure
ACIDOSIS OR ALKALOSIS?

15

BY HANNELORE SWEETWOOD, RN, BS

ALMOST ANY SERIOUS DISEASE or injury can cause respiratory failure either directly or as a secondary effect. Like shock, respiratory failure is frequently a complication of some other problem. But recognizing it is not always easy. You'd readily look for respiratory failure in a patient having an asthmatic attack, or overt pulmonary edema. But in other situations, the onset can be insidious and the symptoms misleading.

Respiratory failure is so perilous you must learn to recognize it in all its forms…and know how to treat it.

What is it?
Respiratory failure is an inability to oxygenate the bloodstream (hypoxemia) or to vent enough waste carbon dioxide (hypercarbia), or both. And what are its effects? Even mild hypoxemia — alone or combined with high CO_2 blood levels — can seriously complicate the patient's clinical condition. Severe respiratory failure, unless promptly detected and corrected, is lethal.

One of the reasons why respiratory failure is so dangerous: The resulting hypoxemia threatens the brain. Although all body cells need oxygen to carry out complete metabolism,

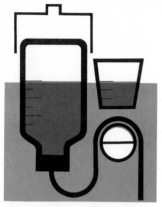

How to interpret lab values
Oxygen tension: The PO_2 represents the oxygen saturation of arterial blood. You need to know the following values for PO_2:
- 80 to 100 mmHg, normal
- 70 mmHg or below, hypoxemia
- 50 mmHg or below, dangerous hypoxemia.

Assuming the patient has no lung disease, giving oxygen greatly increases PO_2. Giving 100% oxygen (when room air is only 21% oxygen) can produce an arterial oxygen tension well above 600 mmHg in a healthy person. So you must take oxygen administration into account when you evaluate the results of blood-gas analysis. Consider, for example, that a patient is receiving oxygen by nasal cannula at a flow rate of 7 liters per minute and his PO_2 is 90 mmHg. Normally, a flow rate of 7 liters per minute of oxygen results in a PO_2 around 200 mmHg. So, if the patient receiving this much oxygen has a PO_2 of only 90 mmHg, you can be sure he has some respiratory insufficiency. Without supplementary oxygen this is in normal range.

Carbon dioxide tension: The PCO_2 is the single best measure of adequacy of alveolar ventilation. You need to know the following values for PCO_2:
- 34 to 46 mmHg, normal;

most tissue cells are capable of sustaining life for varying periods by anaerobic metabolism. (But this process releases large quantities of lactic acid into the bloodstream. Since the lungs in these circumstances cannot vent enough CO_2 to compensate, the result is metabolic acidosis and possibly respiratory acidosis, too.) But brain cells cannot function without oxygen. When the oxygen supply is inadequate, brain cells die and can't be revived even if the body survives. Most vulnerable to hypoxemia are the highest centers of the brain — those that control memory, judgment, and intellect.

With this in mind, you might think that giving oxygen might seem to be the answer each time. But giving some patients plenty of oxygen will only make them worse. You have to give treatment based on clinical findings. But you must base further treatment on the primary indicator, arterial blood gas analysis (ABG). *Obtain an ABG as soon as possible* in all patients with breathing problems.

Know your ABGs

Blood-gas analysis provides the most accurate means of assessing respiratory function; in fact, respiratory failure is often expressed in terms of blood gas values. The tests measure three things: arterial oxygen tension (PO_2); arterial carbon dioxide tension (PCO_2); and pH. Normal arterial oxygen tension (PO_2) is 80 to 100 mmHg, and normal arterial carbon dioxide tension (PCO_2) is 34 to 46 mmHg. Respiratory failure is described as a PO_2 below 50 mmHg; a PCO_2 above 50 mmHg, or both. And, there's a third factor in blood-gas measurements: the pH, or acid-base imbalance. Normally, the body depends on the lungs to throw off carbon dioxide (carbonic acid gas) that metabolism has produced. This helps keep acids from accumulating in the blood. In respiratory failure the lungs are unable to do their share, inclining the patient toward respiratory acidosis. Such acidemia appears in blood-gas analysis as a pH below 7.35.

Clinical clues to respiratory trouble

Naturally, you'll watch for breathing that's too fast or too slow. But also remember that confusion, anxiety, and pugnacity often mean cerebral anoxia, and hypercarbia may be responsible for lethargy and stupor. Also, tachycardia and hypertension are often the first cardiovascular responses to hypoxemia. Whenever you have any doubt about the adequacy of the patient's breathing, inspect his mouth and upper airway carefully to check for obstructing foreign materials. Be sure the obtunded patient's tongue is pulled forward to allow maximum air flow.

Listen. Rhonchi and coarse rales that you can hear without a stethoscope indicate a collection of fluid in the airways. Crowing, croupy noises on inspiration come with obstruction in the upper airways. In older children and adults, grunting expirations may mean the same thing. When bronchial constriction is severe, as in acute asthma, you can hear the wheezes without a stethoscope.

To detect other abnormalities, such as absence of sound over a portion of the lung, you will have to auscultate the chest. If you hear adventitious sounds such as rales, wheezes, and friction rubs, they are apt to mean a serious disorder.

When a patient is using his auxiliary respiratory muscles to breathe, he's likely to need immediate attention. Accessory muscles usually come into play only when all the patient's strength is concentrated on the sheer effort of breathing. But this full use of the respiratory muscles takes a great deal of oxygen — from 30% to 50% of oxygen taken into the body will be used just to drive the overworked respiratory apparatus.

As for *cyanosis,* often described as one of the signs of respiratory failure, it's *a very late sign,* indeed. It indicates not just hypoxemia but dangerous desaturation of arterial blood. Patients may suffer serious ischemic damage to the heart, brain, and kidneys long before you can see cyanosis.

Treatment Varies
There is no single way to treat respiratory failure. Treatment of hypoxia and hypercarbia vary according to the reason for it. Blood-gas findings separate patients with respiratory failure into one of four treatment groups:
1) *PO_2 is below 70 mm Hg and PCO_2 is below 34 mm Hg* (hypoxemia with hyperventilation). In this situation, the lungs are struggling against some obstacle to oxygenate the blood. Give the patient oxygen, selecting method and liter-flow according to degree of hypoxemia. A nasal cannula can be useful for moderate hypoxemia; a non-rebreathing mask, if it's severe. If the work of breathing becomes exhausting to the patient, he may need the assistance of a respirator.

ventilation is adequate
• above 46 mmHg, hypercarbia; hypoventilation
• below 35 mmHg, hypocarbia; hyperventilation.
Acid-base balance: The pH describes the acid-base balance of the bloodstream in terms of its concentration of free hydrogen ions (H^+). The greater their concentration, the more acid the solution and the *lower* the pH. Remember the following values for pH and what they mean:
• 6.8 to 7.00, severe life-threatening acidosis incompatible with life if untreated; immediate intervention required.
• 7.0 to 7.35, acidosis, producing acidemia
• 7.35 to 7.45, normal
• 7.45 to 7.7, alkalosis, producing alkalemia
• 7.7 to 7.8, severe, life-threatening alkalosis; immediate intervention required.
The pH is affected by both metabolic and respiratory factors, as well as by chemical buffering systems in the body (see Chapter 7).

2) *PO₂ is below 70 mmHg and PCO₂ 34 to 46 mmHg* (hypoxemia with normal ventilation). In this situation the lungs are not even trying to overcome the poor oxygenation. Give such a patient oxygen as above. But watch him carefully to be sure his respirations don't fall below the normal rate and depth once the hypoxic drive to breathe is lulled by the extra oxygen.

3) *PO₂ is below 70 mm Hg and PCO₂ above 46 mm Hg* (hypoxemia with hypoventilation). This describes the patient with chronic obstructive lung disease. Give such a patient low-flow oxygen — with a Venturi mask, for example. Use all possible means to stimulate increased ventilation. Encourage coughing and diaphragmatic breathing, and clear airways with suction if necessary. IPPB treatment may improve ventilation. If hypoxemia or hypercarbia are severe, or if the patient doesn't respond, he will need intubation and mechanical ventilation. In an emergency, you can ventilate the patient with an Ambu bag and oxygen until other help arrives.

In patients without chronic lung disease, the hypoxemia is probably from hypoventilation for other reasons such as chest trauma or paralysis. The important part of the treatment for any patient with hypoxemia and hypercarbia is to keep the airway open and assist breathing to restore ventilation.

4) *PO₂ is above 70 mm Hg and PCO₂ is above 46 mm Hg* (near-normal oxygenation with hypoventilation). For this patient, you must maintain an open airway. If he's conscious, encourage him to breathe deeply. If he's unconscious, he may need mechanical ventilation.

By keeping alert, you can detect most of these problems early, and avoid tragic and unnecessary loss of life.

DKA
CORRECTING FLUIDS VITAL

16

BY CAROL ANN GRAMSE, RN, BSN

IN THE UNITED STATES, one in every twenty persons develops diabetes. So, you're certain to care for diabetic patients wherever you happen to practice nursing. Do you know how to recognize and deal with its perilous complication, diabetic ketoacidosis (DKA)? The following case history may give you some helpful insights.

Mrs. Kramer, a 32-year-old beautician, was semi-comatose when admitted to the hospital. Her husband reported she had had the "flu" for 4 days before and had been vomiting. In spite of vomiting, she had continued to drink large quantities of water. She was a known diabetic. At admission, she was comatose, with fast, labored breathing. Her breath had the odor of acetone, and she appeared cachexic. The look of dehydration was striking: Her eyes were deeply sunken, her mouth dry, and her skin loose. She had a weak and rapid pulse, Kussmaul breathing, and hypotension. The laboratory reported: blood sugar, 454 mg per 100 ml; CO_2 11 mEq/L; Cl, 93 mEq/L; Na, 130 mEq/L; K, 7.6 mEq/L; and blood gases: pH, 7.27; PCO_2, 22 mmHg; HCO_3^- 13.5 mEq/L; and, PO_2, 90 mmHg.

Mrs. Kramer was in classic ketoacidosis. Had you been in

the room when she was admitted, would you have quickly suspected what her diagnosis would be? Would you have known how to proceed? What fluid and electrolyte disturbances to expect and what to do about them? Could you have anticipated what treatment would be ordered, so that you could give it promptly? If not, reviewing the material in this chapter may help you become a more effective participant in the management of patients with DKA.

The road to DKA

How did Mrs. Kramer, until recently a healthy young woman, get to be so ill? Let's look at the stages of metabolic change that can bring patients like her to a critical state. Ketoacidosis arrives by a complex process that may occur in someone newly diabetic, or in someone who has had the disease for a long time. It may evolve over a period of weeks or just a few hours, if the diabetes is poorly controlled.

Acute insulin deficiency is the cause and the hallmark of diabetic ketoacidosis. When there is insufficient insulin to promote normal cellular glucose uptake, the body resorts to breaking down proteins and fats to meet its energy requirements. Unless treatment interrupts this deranged metabolic process, a cycle of ketosis, acidosis, tissue breakdown, more ketosis and more acidosis eventually ends in severe dehydration, irreversible coma, and death. What causes such insulin depletion? The patient's failure to take insulin as required or prescribed; or, the presence of stress which increases the body's insulin requirement. Some examples of what can trigger ketoacidosis: infection, trauma, surgery, pregnancy, menstruation, emotional upheavals, and ingesting certain drugs.

The first result of insulin deficiency is hyperglycemia. Only a blood sugar test would pick up this symptomless change. Glycosuria follows. Again, only urinalysis would detect it. But then come some unmistakable symptoms — polydipsia, polyuria (up to 5 or 6 *gallons* a day), and inevitable dehydration, possibly followed by oliguria. During polyuria, electrolyte depletion produces increasing muscle weakness, extreme fatigue and malaise. With the burning of fats for energy, ketones (acetone, betahydroxybutyric acid, and acetoacetic acid) accumulate and appear in the blood and urine. Acidosis begins, stimulates the respiratory center, and Kussmaul breathing follows as compensation. At this stage, the fruity odor of acetone on the breath is unmistakable. The patient may also develop abdominal pain and vomiting. Semi-starvation of the cells now brings hunger and increased food intake, but the patient may lose as much as 30 pounds of body weight nevertheless. Finally, the brain can no longer function under severe dehydration, electrolyte imbalance, and acidosis. Untreated, the patient becomes comatose and may die. When all signs, symptoms, and lab values are put to-gether, little else can be confused with DKA. *Suspect DKA in any patient who is comatose, dehydrated, and in deep, la-bored respiration.*

Diagnostic studies confirm

This condition is essentially unmistakable, so treatment may begin without waiting for laboratory test results. But certain tests are needed to confirm it. Expect to find pH below 7.35, increased serum and urine ketones, decreased sodium and chloride level, elevated BUN (because of dehydration or pro-teolysis), and decreased CO_2 levels — through hyperventila-tion. Changes in blood gases also confirm ketoacidosis. The PCO_2 falls below 35 to 40 mmHg, if the patient is compensating for acidosis with an increased respiratory rate. Hyperpnea may increase the PO_2 beyond the normal limit of 95 mmHg. The bicarbonate (HCO_3^-) level falls below 22 mEq/L. Additional blood tests may include a complete blood count. The hemato-crit and hemoglobin values are usually elevated reflecting hemoconcentration due to dehydration. The white blood cell count is usually elevated due to dehydration, stress, or infec-tion. Laboratory tests may also include enzyme studies: lactic acid dehydrogenase and serum glutamic oxalacetic trans-aminase (to detect acute myocardial infarction); and serum amylase (to detect acute pancreatitis).

Fluid and electrolyte losses

High serum glucose levels produce hyperosmolality of the extracellular fluid. This draws cellular water from the cells into the extracellular fluid to maintain osmotic equilibrium. When the serum glucose concentration reaches 180 mg per 100 ml, glucose begins to spill in the urine (glycosuria). Water excre-tion is also increased since approximately 10 to 20 ml of water is usually needed to excrete each gram of glucose. This pro-duces the polyuria that is characteristic in DKA.

ROAD TO HHNK
(Hyperosmolar Hyperglycemic Non-ketosis)

Risk patients include diabetics not dependent on insulin; patients in their 60s; patients with cardiovascular or renal problems, infection, pancreatic disease, emotional stress, glucocorticoid steroid therapy, extensive burns, hemodialysis, or peritoneal dialysis.

Faulty glucose metabolism:

More glucose supplied than body can handle

Replace water immediately to correct severe dehydration and hyperosmolality. Then begin insulin

HHNK: Hyperglycemic hyperosmolar nonketonic coma

Urinary losses

Hyperosmolality of the extracellular fluid and subsequent glucose diuresis results in urinary loss of sodium, potassium, chloride, phosphate, and bicarbonate. Vomiting may add to their loss, and because sodium combines with ketonic anions, its excretion is further increased.

The renal solute load is also raised by the end-products of fat and protein metabolism. This in turn adds to water loss, since these materials have to be in solution to be excreted. Also, rapid deep respirations characterized by ketoacidosis contribute to the exaggerated insensible loss of water.

Fluid volume decrease can reduce plasma sufficiently to produce hypovolemic shock. The resulting decrease in cerebral perfusion can further depress the respiratory center, despite a pH above 7. If severe, hypovolemia results in decreased renal perfusion. The glomerular filtration rate decreases, resulting in renal retention of sulfates, phosphates, potassium, organic acids, magnesium and nonprotein nitrogen waste products. Therefore, when the fluid volume deficit results in circulatory shock, oliguria appears with the increased serum levels of urea, uric acids, ketones, creatinine, nonprotein nitrogen products, and potassium.

Potassium is released from cells secondary to the movement of hydrogen ions into the cell. Eventually, starvation-damaged cells release protein, potassium, glycogen, water, phosphorus and magnesium resulting in cellular deficits. At this point, serum potassium can rise despite cellular potassium deficit.

Rule out other causes

Some doctors rule out hypoglycemia in comatose diabetics with an intravenous infusion of

Insulin depletion: Hyperglycemia but no fat lipolysis

Increased muscle protein breakdown with increased plasma amino acid levels

Decreased serum glucose utilization; increased hepatic glucose utilization

Hyperglycemia: serum sugar — 1000-3000 mg/100 ml; urine — positive sugar, negative acetone; polyphagia, polydipsia, polyuria; vomiting, diarrhea; CNS dysfunction (areflexia, vestibular dysfunction)

Osmotic pressure diuresis with severe water loss, increased sodium concentration, potassium deficiency

Severe dehydration and plasma hyperosmolality: Urine osmolality 350 mOsm/kg, increased respiration but not Kussmaul's, increased BUN

1 mg glucagon or a 50% dextrose solution (after obtaining a blood sample for a glucose test). The hypoglycemic patient responds to this rapidly, and it does not aggravate ketoacidosis.

Your assessment during the physical examination should include frequent determinations of the state of consciousness, type of respiration, pulse rate, rectal temperature, blood pressure, deep-tendon reflexes, tonicity of eyeballs, condition of skin and mucous membranes, and possible sources of infection. Naturally it includes accurate intake and output records. Watch for change from deep, rapid respirations (Kussmaul breathing) to rapid, shallow, gasping respirations. This change may indicate impaired cerebral blood flow to the respiratory center from hypovolemia and circulatory collapse. A falling blood pH may itself alter respirations.

Fever is probably due to infection, but the temperature is usually below normal in ketoacidosis. The low blood pressure and rapid pulse may result from a fluid volume deficit with circulatory failure. This may also affect the level of consciousness, which decreases with increasing acidosis as well.

Treatment of diabetic acidosis focuses on correcting carbohydrate metabolism and fluid and electrolyte imbalance.

First two hours: Insulin first
Insulin should be given as soon as the diagnosis is made. It can be given several ways. *But only regular insulin should be used. Never the long-acting forms.* The delayed action of lente and NPH insulins makes them ineffective when they are needed, and dangerous later. But remember, hypoglycemic coma should always be ruled out before insulin is given.

Potassium in DKA

After the second stage of treatment, potassium levels are likely to be low because:
- intravenous fluids dilute the plasma;
- improved renal function after correction of fluid volume deficit promotes potassium excretion;
- insulin encourages cellular uptake of potassium while glucose lowers its serum levels;
- cellular glycogenesis uses potassium, further lowering serum levels, and finally,
- potassium moves spontaneously into the cells (higher to lower concentration) to correct the cellular potassium deficit.

So, to prevent muscle flaccidity, rapid and shallow respirations (which replaces Kussmaul's respirations), and weakness, carefully monitor potassium levels and correct deficit as needed. For patients who can eat or drink fluids, foods having a high potassium content or oral K+ supplements offer the easiest replacement. For those who cannot, potassium chloride may be added to the intravenous infusions. The rate of the infusion should not exceed 20 mEq per hour; or 100 mEq per twelve hours. Generally, the treatment goal is to replace 25 to 50 percent of the potassium deficit in the first 24 hours.

Never give concentrated potassium salts directly through intravenous tubing. When adding potassium to I.V. container already hanging, or lying on a counter surface, remember to mix it well in the solution. Potassium is a heavy salt and can settle near the neck of the bottle or plastic bag. Unless you disperse it thoroughly throughout the solution, the patient may get a concentrated dose of potassium with rapid fluid administration and develop cardiac arrest.

Depending on the severity of the coma and the age and size of the patient, the initial insulin dose may range from 10 to 200 units. It can be given intravenously, intramuscularly, or subcutaneously. The total initial dose may be given intramuscularly in two injection sites. In a severely ill patient in shock, it is frequently given intravenously. These large doses of insulin are needed to correct acidosis because an abnormal serum globulin in ketoacidosis antagonizes the action of insulin. But watch for too rapid lowering of the blood sugar level. It causes brain edema with a 100% mortality rate. Consequently, glucose administration becomes part of the treatment, although authorities differ on just when to use it — many give it when blood glucose falls below 250 mg/100 ml, but others prefer to wait 4 to 6 hours after initial treatment when the danger of hypoglycemia is greatest. Some hyperglycemia and glycosuria must be tolerated, lest the patient be thrown into hypoglycemic shock. The patient can shift into insulin shock without regaining consciousness and suffer irreparable brain damage. So, insulin doses need to be modified depending on clinical response and lab results. It seems better to underestimate than overestimate the insulin dose. And small, more frequent doses are always safer than large, less frequent ones.

Fluid replacement critical

Parenteral fluids are given immediately (usually through a CVP line and a peripheral line) in liberal amounts because death in diabetic coma is usually due to dehydration or electrolyte imbalance. Some patients may require 4 to 8 liters of fluid in the first 24 hours. Delay in fluid replacement may also cause acute tubular necrosis. A patient can recover from his stupor and hyperglycemia only to lapse into terminal uremia. So, intravenous *sodium chloride* must be started immediately. The patient in diabetic coma has a water and sodium deficit equal to 10% of his body weight and to 40 g of sodium chloride. Two liters of 0.9 percent saline each containing 154 mEq of sodium and chloride should be given in approximately 2 to 4 hours. After the initial infusion, a hypotonic solution (0.45% saline) containing 77 mEq of sodium may be used since water losses usually exceed electrolyte losses.

Blood, plasma, or a blood volume expander is given if the patient has circulatory collapse. To restore circulatory efficiency in sodium-depletion shock, the combination of saline solution and colloids is more effective than either alone.

Potassium levels are usually normal or elevated on admission because dehydration and acidosis force potassium into the blood. As a result, the cells are in potassium deficit even though the serum shows hyperkalemia. Unless potassium levels are carefully monitored, treatment may produce hypokalemia, with muscle weakness or paralysis following. The weakness may fatally affect respiratory and cardiac function. To avoid it, remember that insulin carries extracellular potassium back into the cells along with glucose; and administration of fluids not containing potassium produces hemodilution. Potassium infusion usually begins 4 hours after admission and requires EKG and urinary output monitoring.

Sodium bicarbonate or sodium lactate is given to seriously ill patients with low pH. So you should have supplies of sodium bicarbonate on hand for emergency use. The goal of replacement therapy is to raise pH to 7.2, but no higher than 7.4. Bicarbonate therapy is usually considered when CO_2 levels fall to 8 mEq/L. However, bicarbonate may cause the patient's sensorium to worsen. This is attributed to a higher hydrogen concentration in the cerebrospinal fluid that results from the more rapid transfer of carbon dioxide than of bicarbonate to the spinal fluid. For this reason, using bicarbonate in DKA is now controversial. Most authorities have routinely used bicarbonate in large amounts to correct metabolic acidosis. But others contend that bicarbonate actually raises the carbonic acid level, enhances cerebral acidosis, and may prolong diabetic coma. Many now feel that correction with insulin and I.V. fluids containing electrolytes and glucose is sufficient and allows the kidney and lungs to correct acidosis in a more physiologic way.

Second to sixth hours: Stabilize insulin and fluid. After the initial insulin dosage, monitor urine sugar and acetone levels hourly and give additional insulin accordingly. Frequently, clinical improvement occurs while acetonuria remains strongly positive. So, both the clinical factors and urine acetone concentration help determine insulin dosages. In adults, after one to three doses of insulin, reduction in urine glucose and acetone levels usually permits lowering the insulin dose to 5 units for each "plus" of urine glucose.

Rarely, "insulin resistance" occurs in patients who normally need up to 200 units insulin daily, causing a delayed response to ketoacidosis treatment. Or, allergy to the standard preparation of insulin (beef and pork are sources) may develop and another form of insulin would then be indicated. But the most common cause of delayed response to insulin is obesity. Obese patients may need up to 100 units daily and may resist standard doses for acidosis.

During this phase of treatment the fluid and electrolyte imbalances in ketoacidosis may be corrected with several kinds of solutions. Another liter of isotonic saline can be given over a period of 2 to 3 hours. If the patient develops hyperventilation, extreme acidosis, or a low carbon dioxide content (<8 mEq/L), sodium lactate and bicarbonate solution can be used. After electrolyte replacement, solutions of 5% dextrose or fructose in water usually replace water deficits. Be sure to monitor total fluid intake. Adjust the rate of infusion so total fluid intake does not exceed 5,000 ml. Consider severe volume deficit corrected if, after infusion of 3,000 ml of fluid, urinary output exceeds 40 ml per hour (normal range is 30 to 60 ml per hour). Ideally, 50 to 80 percent of the patient's lost water, chloride, and sodium should be replaced within the first 24 hours. At this stage, oral fluid intake should not exceed 100 to 120 ml per hour for adults. If nausea occurs, withhold oral fluids for another 2 to 6 hours. Taking another history may now be appropriate. Since a now alert and cooperative patient may provide more information and, since severe dehydration has been corrected, significant physical findings which were masked by fluid loss may become apparent.

Six to twenty-four hours

Continue to obtain serum glucose and carbon dioxide determinations every 4 to 6 hours. Adjust insulin dosages according to glucose findings and to urinary acetone reports. At this stage, oral feedings may begin — usually with carbohydrate intake under 10 g per hour and soft or liquid food such as oatmeal, gruel, orange juice, or mild diluted Half-and-Half with water. If the patient cannot tolerate these, continue intravenous glucose (5 to 10 percent dextrose in saline) at approximately 200 ml per hour. Continue to monitor serum electrolyte levels every 8 to 12 hours. After the second day, the doctor will start intermediate-acting insulin and appropriate diet. At this stage, review management of diabetes. Try to suggest preventive measures.

Abdominal Surgery
FLUID AND ELECTROLYTE COMPLICATIONS

17

BY JOYCE KEE, RN, BSN, MSN

IF YOU OFTEN CARE for surgical patients, you know how quickly their fluid and electrolyte status can change — within hours or even minutes — often in the doctor's absence. Then, it's up to you to recognize the change, evaluate it correctly, and take appropriate action.

To manage such problems correctly, your assessment begins the moment the patient enters your care. You can recognize imbalances more promptly if you learn to anticipate the most likely ones. To do so, you need to know the patient's preexisting and present health problems, his symptoms, his renal function and electrolyte balance.

Watch for fluid and electrolyte imbalance and report the first signs of it. Check all laboratory findings as soon as they become available. Are they within normal limits? If not, let the doctor know right away. Watch for signs of dehydration: thirst, dry skin, dry mucous membranes, low grade fever, increased pulse rate, oliguria, and increased BUN and hemoglobin. Report these signs promptly so that dehydration can be corrected before surgery. Remember, careful assessment *before* surgery can help avoid complications *after* surgery. This was certainly true in Tom Piccola's case.

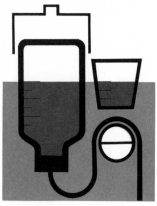

What to know
Here are some important
questions to answer about your
patient before he undergoes
surgery.
  ● What are the patient's
preexisting health problems?
  ● Does he have a cardiovascular
problem?
  ● Was edema present on
admission?
  ● Did the patient have problems
that might lead to dehydration,
vomiting, diarrhea, anorexia,
diaphoresis, or hyperventilation?
  ● How old is the patient? The
very old and the very young are
exceedingly vulnerable and need
close assessment.
  ● What is the patient's fluid
output? If it's less than 500 ml per
day, he may be dehydrated or
may have renal insufficiency.
  ● Were laboratory tests ordered?
If so, monitor serum electrolytes,
hemoglobin, hematocrit, BUN,
and creatinine.

Tom Piccola, a 55-year-old accountant, was hospitalized because of vomiting and abdominal pain that had persisted for 3 days. He had a 10-year history of diverticulitis. During past flare-ups, omitting roughage and gas-forming foods would relieve his symptoms, but had not helped this time. At admission, his skin and mucous membranes were dry and skin turgor was poor. His vital signs were: temperature, 37.7° C. (99.9° F.); pulse, 94; respiration, 30. His laboratory results were: K, 3.2 mEq/L; Na, 134 mEq/L; Cl, 96 mEq/L; BUN, 35 mg/100 ml; and Hgb, 18.5 g. Mr. Piccola's clinical symptoms, physical assessment, and laboratory findings indicated dehydration.

To correct his fluid and electrolyte deficit, 2 liters of 5% dextrose in 0.45% saline and 2 liters of 5% dextrose in 0.2% saline with KCl (20 mEq/L) were ordered for the first 24 hours. He was scheduled for gastrointestinal surgery the next day. During surgery and immediately afterward, Mr. Piccola received 3 more liters of 5% dextrose in water. Nursing assessment for fluid and electrolyte changes continued. He received 2 liters of 5% dextrose in water and 2 liters of 5% dextrose in 0.45% sodium chloride daily. Later, he was watched carefully for fluid deficit, especially between the second and fifth postoperative day (when a spontaneous diuresis usually occurs). Because Mr. Piccola had a Miller-Abbott tube connected to suction, he was losing sodium, bicarbonate and some potassium. So, his electrolytes were monitored closely. On the first postoperative day, his laboratory results were: K, 3.5 mEq/L; Na, 132 mEq/L; and Cl, 96 mEq/L. His serum potassium was within normal range but could drop if supplemental KCl was not given. When blood gases were drawn 10 hours after surgery, the results were: pH, 7.34; Pco_2, 50 mmHg; HCO_3^-, 24 mEq/L. He was hypoventilating and said that breathing deeply was painful.

Mr. Piccola was retaining CO_2 in excess and was developing mild respiratory acidosis. The doctor prescribed meperidine HCl (Demerol) 50 mg q 4 h, p.r.n., to relieve pain, even though narcotics tend to depress respiration. In this case, they helped normalize respiration by allowing the patient to breathe normally without pain. He continued to improve. His recovery was uneventful and he was discharged after 7 days.

Consider the surgery
The patient who has gastrointestinal surgery is apt to lose

electrolytes in amounts sufficient to cause imbalance. Potassium, hydrogen, and chloride are concentrated in the stomach; sodium and bicarbonate, in the intestine. So, the patient who's been vomiting or is on suction is losing potassium, hydrogen, and chloride. These losses make him vulnerable to hypokalemia and alkalosis.

After surgery

Expect and watch for two derangements that typically follow surgery: fluid and acid-base imbalances. Let's look at fluid imbalances first. These are common after surgery when the patient is allowed only sips of water or ice chips, and is receiving intravenous infusions of dextrose and water.

Water intoxication develops because of the body's normal response to surgical trauma. Immediately after surgery, urinary output declines. Renal retention of water in excess of sodium increases the extracellular fluid, causing hypotonicity. Osmosis then causes fluid to accumulate in the cells, a condition called water intoxication. It's aggravated if the patient drinks copious amounts of liquids postoperatively, while receiving intravenous dextrose solution. Cerebral cells frequently are affected first. Watch for these symptoms of water intoxication: headache, sweating, flushed and hot skin, behavioral changes, incoordination, and drowsiness. Report them promptly.

Edema is retention of a different sort, a shift of fluid to the site of injured or infected tissues. Edema also results from cardiac insufficiency, a more worrisome development. Watch for it in patients with impaired cardiac function who are receiving intravenous fluids in quantity. Watch for coughing, dyspnea, neck-vein enlargement, swelling of the extremities, and anasarca (generalized massive edema) — all signs of overhydration (hypervolemia).

Dehydration, too, can occur right after surgery, either because of blood loss or inadequate fluid intake. Also, it can occur between the second and fifth postoperative day due to diuresis. This diuresis is considered normal, yet the loss should be assessed. So, check the patient's chart for urinary output, estimated blood loss, and I.V. fluid infused.

Shock, it goes without saying, is evidence of severe fluid disturbance, the consequence of heavy blood loss (hypovolemia). Such losses may lead to renal insufficiency.

So, watch for rising pulse rate which can indicate impending shock or hypovolemia. Falling blood pressure is often a late symptom of shock (see Chapter 18).

Next, anticipate acid-base imbalances. These are the conditions apt to precipitate them:

• *Hyperventilation* causes respiratory alkalosis. This commonly develops in the seriously ill, gripped by anxiety. When hyperventilating patients blow off too much carbon dioxide this, in time, causes *respiratory alkalosis*. Early symptoms — rapid shallow breathing, vertigo, and rosy complexion — are eventually followed by signs of tetany as increased alkalinity of extracellular fluid causes decreased ionization of calcium. In respiratory alkalosis, serum CO_2 and PCO_2 are depressed; the pH, elevated. The condition can be corrected if the patient can be made to breathe slowly and deeply.

• *Hypoventilation* develops when anesthetics, narcotic analgesics, sedatives, or pain depress respiration. An inadequate exchange of gases results in CO_2 retention and, hence, respiratory acidosis. Serum CO_2 and PCO_2 are elevated; pH, depressed or close to normal. Again deep breathing corrects; breathing exercises sometimes help.

• *Vomiting or gastric intubation* causes the loss of hydrogen and chloride as well as that highly important cation, potassium. With loss of hydrogen and chloride ions, the patient develops *metabolic alkalosis*. The serum CO_2 and pH are elevated. Fluid replacement with one-half normal saline and KCl helps to correct metabolic alkalosis. Later, metabolic alkalosis can shift into metabolic acidosis due to cellular breakdown and accumulation of acid metabolites (lactic acid).

• *Diarrhea and intestinal intubation* can cause excessive loss of alkaline intestinal secretions, bile, and pancreatic juice. Lost are sodium and potassium along with bicarbonate, which is normally plentiful in the intestine. Bicarbonate loss causes *metabolic acidosis*. The serum CO_2 and pH will be depressed. Fluid replacement with bicarbonate helps correct this.

Summing up then, your role in assessment, intervention, and evaluation of fluid and electrolyte changes in postoperative patients includes: reporting abnormal electrolyte findings; observing for signs and symptoms of hypervolemia or hypovolemia and electrolyte imbalance; determining urinary status; noting nonmeasured fluid losses as from diaphoresis; and recognizing changes in acid-base balance.

Shock
FLUIDS RESTORE CIRCULATION

18

BY MINNIE ROSE, RN, BSN, MEd

HYPOVOLEMIC SHOCK...septic shock...cardiogenic shock ...each presents its own special problems. The quicker you recognize them — and act — the better the patient's chances of survival.

Classic symptoms late

The body can compensate for a 10% blood loss so efficiently — by constriction of the arteriolar bed, increased heart rate, force of contraction, and fluid redistribution — that vital signs, skin color, and skin temperature remain normal. Only the cardiac output will be slightly reduced. But by the time blood loss reaches 15% to 25%, cardiac output will be markedly decreased, and classic signs of shock will have appeared. At this point, the patient's condition will be unstable and his shock (which may have been prevented if treatment had started at 10% blood loss) will increasingly resist treatment.

So, anticipate shock in any condition where it's a likely complication: in anaphylaxis; anoxia; any condition associated with fluid loss or sequestered fluid (third space); heart failure from any cause; major obstruction of blood flow; any severe infection; and endocrine and metabolic disorders. Be

Classification of shock

If you classify shock in two different groups — cardiogenic or central, and peripheral — you may understand its dynamics more easily. Cardiogenic shock refers to those cases resulting from dysfunction of the heart itself. An impairment in cardiac emptying or filling can lead to shock.

Peripheral shock encompasses those cases of hypovolemia or of pooling of blood in the capillaries, as in patients with hemorrhage or septicemia.

Remember — more than one single condition may precipitate shock. Others may aggravate the situation, creating a vicious circle. So your understanding of shock and all its facets is vital to your patient's care.

		DEFINITION	PHYSIOLOGICAL DISTURBANCES	ETIOLOGY
CARDIOGENIC (central)		Primary insufficiency of cardiac output due to impaired pumping action	Myocardial	myocardial infarction, acute myocarditis, terminal failure
			Valvular	rupture of valve cusp
		Secondary insufficiency due to filling defect	Mechanical	pulmonary embolism, pericardial tamponade, valvular obstruction by atrial tumor, or thrombus
			Functional	ectopic-tachycardias, severe arrhythmias
PERIPHERAL		Decreased blood volume; hypovolemia	Hemogenic (loss of blood)	hemorrhage
			Traumatic (loss of plasma)	burns or trauma
			Dehydration	loss of fluids via kidneys gastrointestinal tract sweat glands
		Pooling of blood	Endotoxic (septic)	bacterial or viral infection
			Anaphylactic	histamine or histamine-like substance
			Neurogenic (reflex or neurohumoral)	pain drugs (anesthesia, soporifics), heat stroke

ready to start treatment at the first signs of shock — for example, the quick pulse and the clammy skin. *Watch for the following early warning signs:*

• *Skin changes* (temperature and color) reflect tissue oxygenation and perfusion. Continuing cold clammy skin during fluid replacement signals continuing peripheral vascular constriction — an indication for faster fluid administration. In such patients, crystalloids must be given rapidly to prevent fluid from diffusing into the interstitial space as fast as it is administered. When treating shock, fluids are generally given rapidly and then slowed. Flushing and sweating indicate overheating — a condition which increases metabolic rate and the need for oxygen. Continuing pallor and cyanosis in a shock patient generally indicate tissue hypoxia, but cyanosis in the lips and nail beds may only mean that the patient is cold. To avoid confusion, check for cyanosis in an extremity that is lightly covered. And since *change is the key,* the evaluation for color should be made by the same person each time. In dark-skinned patients, use the soles and palms for evaluation. But remember that good skin color is not proof of adequate tissue oxygenation. Some patients look pink with dangerously low oxygen levels.

• *Blood pressure and pulse:* Rapid pulse may be the first sign of shock, whereas, a drop in blood pressure is often a *late* sign. Eventually systolic pressure drops 30 mmHg or more.

• *Respiration* becomes rapid and shallow. Such air hunger is a common early sign of shock as the body tries to compensate for tissue hypoxia. Slow breathing — 2 to 3 breaths per minute — appears late in shock after failure of the compensatory mechanisms.

• *Temperature* usually drops below normal with hemorrhagic shock. Again, watch for

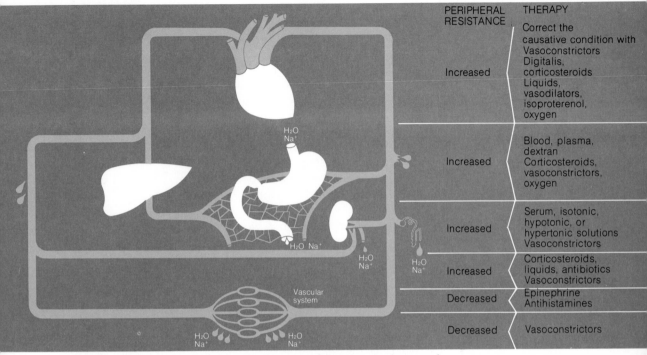

	PERIPHERAL RESISTANCE	THERAPY
	Increased	Correct the causative condition with Vasoconstrictors Digitalis, corticosteroids Liquids, vasodilators, isoproterenol, oxygen
	Increased	Blood, plasma, dextran Corticosteroids, vasoconstrictors, oxygen
	Increased	Serum, isotonic, hypotonic, or hypertonic solutions Vasoconstrictors
	Increased	Corticosteroids, liquids, antibiotics Vasoconstrictors
	Decreased	Epinephrine Antihistamines
	Decreased	Vasoconstrictors

change: Gradually rising temperature may signal developing sepsis.

• *Restlessness* is common in early shock and indicates hypoxia. If restlessness continues despite oxygen administration, it is probably the result of fear and pain. Your reassurance can go a long way toward relieving fear. Relieving pain can be more difficult, since most narcotics depress respiratory function. If narcotics are needed, they are usually given intravenously at one-third the normal IM dose.

• *Urine output* below 30 ml per hour signals marked reduction in renal blood flow — a sign of severe shock. Anytime you notice a pattern of decreasing urine output and hypovolemia, increase fluid infusion rate to the maximum and call a doctor.

Whatever the cause of shock, the end result is reduced circulation, tissue hypoperfusion, and body cell deprivation of oxygen and nutrients. And so, treatment aims to correct the underlying cause and to increase tissue perfusion. Sometimes the underlying cause is obvious and easily corrected. For example, in hemorrhagic shock, blood replacement will usually restore circulatory homeostasis if the duration of shock has not been too long. In insulin shock, treatment with glucose will restore circulation. Let's look at the treatment of shock in order of priority.

First, ensure ventilation

At the first sign of shock, ensure an open airway, draw blood for blood-gas determination, and start oxygen. Do not attempt assessment of respiratory competence on appearance alone. Remember, cyanosis is a late sign. And many patients look pink and comfortable with a PO_2 of

Drugs commonly used in shock
Corticosteroids: dexamethasone
   (Decadron, Hexadrol),
   hydrocortisone
*Positive inotropic/
chromotrophics:*
   isoproterenol (Isuprel),
   dopamine hydrochloride
   (Intropin)
Digitalis glycosides: ouabain,
   digoxin (Lanoxin), deslanoside
   (Cedilanid-D)
Vasopressors: levarterenol
   bitartrate (Levophed),
   epinephrine (Adrenalin),
   metaraminol (Aramine)
Anticoagulant: heparin
Systemic buffers: tromethamine
   (THAM), sodium bicarbonate,
   sodium lactate
Antihistamine: diphenhydramine
   (Benadryl)
Spasmolytic: aminophylline

45 to 50 — a level at which arrhythmias become likely.

The serum pH may be deceptive. The PCO_2 is the key to detecting compensatory acidosis. A low PCO_2 in the presence of a low pH and low bicarbonate level indicates that the respiratory system is compensating (normal PCO_2 is 34 to 46 mmHg). A rising PCO_2 with a persistently low pH and low bicarbonate levels is a warning that the respiratory compensatory mechanism is failing, usually because the patient has become exhausted. To prevent respiratory failure in such patients, use a volume respirator to remove excess carbon dioxide; oxygen alone is useless at this stage.

Start fluid replacement
How to restore blood volume? The rule of thumb is: *Replace whatever has been lost.* In traumatic shock, give blood and crystalloids; in septic shock, give plasma, dextran, and salt solutions (if the hematocrit is over 35%); and in cardiogenic shock, give crystalloids and vasodilators. Most authorities recommend infusing 5% dextrose in water or a balanced salt solution while the patient's needs are being assessed.

Then, as soon as possible, *begin measuring the central venous pressure (CVP)* or pulmonary artery pressure. These are important guidelines for fluid replacement (or restriction, in some cases). Because fluid needs fluctuate widely and often quickly in the shock patient, and because you must replace volume as quickly as you can without overloading the heart, central monitoring is necessary.

How to assess the competency of the heart? Because peripheral blood pressure is often unreliable, or even undetectable because of decrease in peripheral resistance, direct arterial monitoring of blood pressure is becoming standard practice. However, if intra-arterial pressure systems are unavailable, palpation of the femoral artery is more reliable than the radial and brachial for taking a shock patient's pulse. Palpation also tells the quality of the pulse, which the monitors cannot provide. A thready pulse indicates low blood pressure, and perhaps the need for volume replacement but may also occur in overload.

Monitor medications
Naturally, treatment depends on the cause of shock. Drugs are used in its treatment mainly to alter peripheral resistance — by

increasing or decreasing it. There is much controversy over which approach to use. Those who advocate increasing peripheral resistance (with vasopressors) believe that arterial pressure must be maintained to ensure adequate tissue perfusion. Those who recommend vasodilators for shock hold an opposite view. They believe that decreased arterial pressure is a symptom, not a cause of shock, and that raising arterial pressure makes tissue perfusion more difficult. So, they use vasodilators to increase cardiac output and improve tissue perfusion. Also controversial is the use of steroids. Some experts say they have no beneficial effect whatever; others say they reduce mortality significantly. Your main nursing problems with drugs in treating shock involve the management of hypotension.

Promote rest

Shock patients have very little energy reserve, and so it is important to *allow the patient to rest* and relieve his discomfort and apprehension. Pain exhausts the patient and can deepen shock, so pain relief is important indeed. Unfortunately, it is also difficult. Most sedatives and analgesics depress respiration, so full doses cannot be given. And because circulation is poor, intramuscular injections do not provide reliable relief, and can cause toxic effects when circulation is restored. For these reasons, one-third to one-half of the usual I.M. dose of prescribed analgesic is usually given intravenously for pain relief.

Watch for complications

The patient in shock must lie inert for several hours to days, a situation conducive to decubiti, respiratory depression, and circulatory problems. So, do not overlook ordinary measures to improve circulation (turning or tilting the patient every 2 hours; deep breathing and coughing; exercising the arms and legs; and gentle rubbing of the patient's skin to increase circulation). Keep the patient warm. Allowing him to become too chilly, or to become too warm (from heating pads or too many blankets) can adversely affect peripheral circulation.

Very little *can't* go wrong in shock so you must constantly reassess such a patient for significant change. But one complication is both common and often fatal — adult respiratory distress syndrome (ARDS). This syndrome has replaced renal

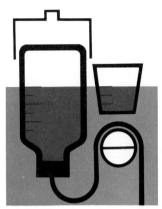

Precautions for drugs used in shock
When using
- *Corticosteroids:* Watch for GI bleeding.
- *Isuprel:* Monitor EKG with defibrillator at bedside. Slow or stop infusion if heart rate exceeds 110/minute. Measure urine output and BP every 15 minutes. Do not use with epinephrine.
- *Intropin:* Monitor EKG for ventricular arrhythmias. Maintain CVP at 10 to 15 cm H_2O. Check urine output every 30 minutes. Do not add to alkaline solutions.
- *Digitalis:* Monitor pulse and EKG constantly.
- *Vasopressors:* Monitor EKG for PVCs. Watch for ventricular decompensation and pulmonary edema. Stop if headache, chest pain, nausea, or hypotension develops.
- *Heparin:* Monitor with partial thromboplastin times (PTT). Maintain at 2½ times control.
- *Systemic buffers:* Give slowly. Monitor EKG.
- *Aminophylline:* Give slowly.

failure as the major complication leading to death from shock. Three things make it more likely: overaggressive fluid therapy, microemboli, and superinfection. ARDS is pulmonary failure (including pulmonary congestion, hemorrhage, edema, and shunting) that follows successful resuscitation from hypotension and develops anywhere from 1 to 6 days after treatment of shock. The patient looks deceptively well, but begins to hyperventilate and becomes progressively dyspneic with rapid shallow breathing, a productive cough, elevated PCO_2, and low PO_2. Current treatment includes ventilatory support with positive end-expiratory pressure (PEEP), oxygen, diuretics, heparin, and steroids. There is a high mortality rate with ARDS.

When skin color returns

As vital signs return to normal and the skin becomes warm and rosy, continue to watch urine output carefully. Continuing oliguria (less than 30 ml per hour) indicates impending kidney failure, and you must inform the doctor immediately. If urine output is good and the patient appears stable, slowly withdraw support, continuing to monitor at regular frequent intervals.

Medical opinion differs on many aspects of treating shock, so nursing practice differs from one hospital to another. But one aspect remains constant: the critical need for continuous assessment — watching for the earliest signs of change in the quantity of circulating fluids and the degree of tissue perfusion. Your skill at such assessment and at correcting whatever abnormalities you may find is a critical factor in the patient's recovery.

Burns
FLUIDS RESUSCITATE

19

BY CLAUDELLA ARCHAMBEAULT JONES, RN
AND KATHRYN E. RICHARDS, MD

IN THE FIRST FEW DAYS after a severe burn, the patient's major problems come from changes in fluid and electrolyte status. The doctor prescribes fluid resuscitation for such patients, but the amount actually given each hour is a nursing decision based on hourly urine output and other factors. To care for burned patients, you need to know how fluid resuscitation works. Your patient's survival will depend on it. Tom Parker's case was typical.

Tom Parker, a 54-year-old welder, was admitted to the hospital with serious burns after an industrial explosion. He had partial and full-thickness burns over 40% of his body including his head, neck, arms, back, and the back of both legs.

At admission, his respirations were 22 and regular. His blood gases were normal, and he was having no respiratory distress. But his head and neck burns could soon cause oropharyngeal and laryngeal edema, so we inserted an endotracheal tube. He was hypotensive with a systolic pressure of 90, monitored by palpation. Auscultation was already difficult because edema of the arms and legs obscured BP sounds.

To counteract burn shock we began aggressive fluid therapy

immediately. We inserted a subclavian catheter, drew baseline lab values, and started a liter of lactated Ringer's solution. We used a formula as a guideline: e.g., 4 ml x 102.1 (kg body weight) x 40 (% of burn) for a total of 16,336 ml. This patient would need no more than this total. For the first 3 hours postburn he received 1000 ml per hour but, due to his sound cardiovascular system and no history of renal problems, his output soon stabilized at 50 ml/hour. The I.V. was slowed correspondingly so that he received a total of 5900 ml in the first 8 hours.

We monitored blood pressure, pulse rate, and respirations every 15 minutes for one hour, and then hourly; and temperature every hour. We also checked Tom's central venous pressure (CVP) hourly to assess blood volume. We inserted a Foley catheter to allow hourly urine measurements and analyses to give us an early indication if renal failure developed. After getting a pertinent history, we gave tetanus toxoid (0.5 ml I.M.) and began wound care.

We positioned him with his arms elevated above the level of the heart and lungs to reduce edema of the arms and workload of the cardiovascular system.

We connected the endotracheal tube to a respirator, and gave warmed humidified oxygen at 80% concentration. We inserted a nasogastric tube for decompression and removal of gastric contents and gave Maalox, 30 ml, every 2 hours. A chest X-ray was done to check the lungs for any abnormalities and to check placement of the endotracheal tube, and subclavian catheter (CVP line). Tom's urine was analyzed for sugar/acetone, protein, pH and specific gravity. The hematocrit — measured on admission and every 6 hours during initial replacement — is another guide to titration. Because of the shift of water from the bloodstream to the tissues during burn shock, the hematocrit is elevated at first, but with adequate fluid replacement, it falls back to normal. Tom's was normal on the third day postburn. After 5 days, Tom's urinary output suddenly increased signaling the successful completion of the emergent period.

Why are fluids so important?

With severe burn injury, the inflammatory process in the first 24 to 48 hours shifts huge amounts of fluids out of the blood into interstitial spaces. It does so because increased capillary

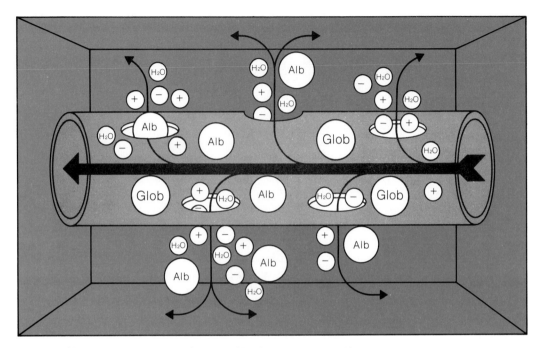

permeability upsets the osmosis and diffusion that normally maintain a delicate balance. This shift is called burn shock. Untreated, it can lead to hypovolemic shock and death. Fluid therapy is needed to preserve circulation. It is needed immediately and should always precede local treatment of the burn itself.

Fluid therapy is so important to the immediate care of the severely burned patient, that the need for it actually defines the emergent period — the first few days postburn when first aid is given; when the severity of the burn is determined; and when the foundation is laid for future care. The emergent period ends when the patient's condition stabilizes, fluids return to the vascular space, diuresis occurs, and he no longer needs intensive fluid therapy. How soon this happens depends greatly on good nursing care, particularly on the nurse's skill with fluid treatment.

Fluids restore cardiac output. Your primary goal of fluid replacement is to restore cardiac output — depressed mostly because of volume deficit. This is approximately proportional to the extent and depth of injury, and is greatest during the first 12 hours. It lasts for 18 to 24 hours after a severe burn, and

A vital loss
Burn damage increases capillary permeability. This increase and the inflammatory process cause leakage into the interstitial space. Since water, electrolyte, and albumin molecules are small, a greater number of them are lost from the vascular space than of blood cells (red, white, and platelets) or of large protein molecules like globulins, which remain in the vessels.

calls for rapid administration of resuscitation fluid.

Who needs fluids? Anyone with a full-thickness burn greater than 20% of his body, and any burned patient younger than 4 or older than 35, or with complicating factors: dehydration, hemorrhage, or other injuries.

What kinds of fluids? Fluid therapy replaces the fluid leaving the vascular space — primarily water, electrolytes, and albumin. The major portion of the fluid is given in the form of an isotonic-balanced buffer electrolyte solution, with albumin. Lactated Ringer's solution (with or without albumin) is usually the fluid of choice during resuscitation after burns. It is chosen because it has an electrolyte balance similar to that of the blood; colloids such as albumin may be added to help maintain osmotic pressure, but not everyone agrees that it is helpful in the first 24 hours. But authorities do believe it reduces colloid extravasation which pulls along water, if not in the first 24 hours, then provenly in the second 24 hours.

Lactated Ringer's solution is a balanced salt solution with a composition close to that of extracellular fluid, except for a slight difference in the amount of sodium. (It contains 154 mEq/L.) The lactate gets rapidly converted in the body to bicarbonate, and the acidosis of burn shock disappears within 12 to 24 hours after injury.

How much fluid? Titration maintains urinary output at a predetermined level by carefully measured fluid volume replacement. It requires the close monitoring of...

• I.V. fluids and any oral intake. (Any burn greater than 20% total body surface area [TBSA] causes a decrease in fluid to splanchnic organs, which results in decreased gastrointestinal mobility and ileus. These patients receive nothing by mouth and may require nasogastric drainage until bowel sounds return.)

• all output

• vital signs (blood pressure, pulse rate, arterial O_2 saturation, central venous pressure

• sometimes, pulmonary artery wedge pressure

• hematocrit

• weight (compared to preburn weight)

Many formulas are available for calculating fluid replacement, but the one most often used is the Baxter formula: 4.0 ml per kg body weight times percentage of total body surface area burned, up to 50%, with one half given in the first 8 hours; one fourth in the second 8 hours; and one fourth in the third 8 hours.

Fluid replacement requirements may go as high as 1000 ml per hour in the first few hours but gradually taper off. *Rarely are more than 10,000 ml given in 24 hours,* and then only in a very large adult, but this is uncommon! This enormous volume of fluids seems unbelievably large to nurses used to caring for patients who need only maintenance fluids. Remember that a formula is only an *estimate* of fluid needs and a starting point. The patient's clinical response is a more accurate guide to the amount needed. The formula cannot take into account the patient's cardiovascular status, past medical history, renal status, and respiratory involvement — all very serious considerations. For example: a patient who sustained face and neck injury, or was burned in an enclosed space such as in an explosion, will likely have upper and possible lower airway involvement. Fluid therapy for this patient would be on the dry side to prevent extravasation of fluids in the lungs, increased pulmonary edema, and stiff, wet lungs, leading to shunting, severe pulmonary problems and congestive heart failure!

Daily weights essential

Accurate, nude, daily weights are essential for evaluating fluid therapy in severely burned patients. Such patients receive nothing by mouth; thus all weight gain is fluid. One liter of fluid (1000 ml) equals a kilogram (2.2 lb). The patient should gain *no more than 15% of his normal body weight* during initial fluid therapy. For instance, a patient who weighed 100 lb preburn should gain no more than 15 lb (retention of approximately 7 liters of fluid, after output and obligatory insensible loss). Obviously, this much fluid in the interstitial spaces or returning to vascular space risks overload, congestive failure, or pulmonary edema.

• *How much urine output?* For adults in previously good health, desirable output often ranges between 30 to 60 ml of urine an hour; for children or the elderly, 10 to 30 ml per hour. Infants, and patients with cardiac, respiratory, or renal problems, require even smaller outputs.

CAUTION! Don't overload fluids. Trying to maintain high urinary output risks fluid overload, increased cardiac output, increased interstitial edema, congestive heart failure, wet lung syndrome (ARDS), and renal failure.

What you must know — fast
The following lab information will help you assess tissue perfusion, electrolyte and acid-base states, the need for sodium bicarbonate, and the patient's response to treatment.
VENOUS BLOOD:
  hematocrit
  protein
  electrolytes (Na, K, Cl, HCO_3^-)
  CO_2
  pH
  PO_2
  urea (BUN)
URINARY OUTPUT:
  Na, K, and Cl concentration
  specific gravity
  protein
  sugar and acetone
  pH
  color
  blood

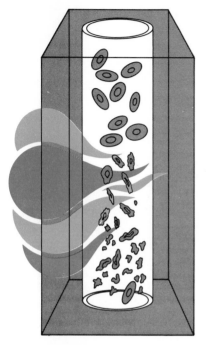

Cell damage too
Patients with severe burns suffer
not only from tissue damage but
also from hemolysis, the
destruction of red blood cells.
These cells release hemoglobin
pigment into the blood. Since the
accumulation of this pigment can
permanently damage the renal
tubules, hemolytic patients
should be treated with fluids and a
diuretic to clear the kidneys as
rapidly as possible.

Although burn formulas help gauge the approximate amount
of fluid replacement needed, accurate fluid replacement depends not only on correct monitoring, but also on accurate
estimation of the size of the burn and on the patient's general
condition. Regardless, hourly monitoring of output and vital
signs to tailor the fluid therapy to the patient is critical to
effective treatment. Adequate hourly urine output indicates
adequate renal blood flow. So careful monitoring of urine
output is necessary because it actually reflects cardiac output.
Remember, IV fluids also leak out of capillaries in burn shock
and the interstitial spaces act as huge sponge! It is especially
easy to overload a child, infant, or elderly person. Their bodies
just cannot compensate for large amounts of fluid.

• *If urinary output is inadequate:* The most common reason
for decreased urinary output in burned patients is that the
calculated amount of fluid replacement is behind schedule.
The second most common reason is that the extent of burn has
been underestimated. To avoid errors, keep fluid on schedule,
watch for improperly running I.V., and for a plugged urinary
catheter!

Deep tissue injury or electrical injury releases free hemoglobin and myoglobin from blood and muscle cells, resulting in
hemo-myoglobinemia and hemoglobinuria. Passage of this de-
stroyed cell tissue throughout the basement membrane of the
glomerulus will plug the renal tubules; untreated, it will result
in acute tubular necrosis (ATN). Its outward sign is black
urine. At the first sign of black urine, the doctor will order
mannitol (Osmitrol), an osmotic diuretic, to flush the kidneys.
Hemoglobinuria clears dramatically if treated early. With only
two doses of mannitol and increased fluids to replace the
diuresis, the urine may clear within a few hours.

• *Consider potassium and other electrolytes:* Damaged cells
pour out their stores of potassium, but this rarely causes
persistent measurable hyperkalemia, except in the massive
injuries such as electrical. In most burns, initial *hyper*kalemia
soon shifts to *hypo*kalemia.

After the shock phase, in about 36 to 48 hours, the interstitial fluids reenter the blood stream producing hemodilution.
As diuresis begins, the sodium and other electrolytes return to
the vascular spaces, and the potassium is wasted (secondary
to some element of acute tubular necrosis and, in part, to
aldosterone and other hormonal influences). This phase may

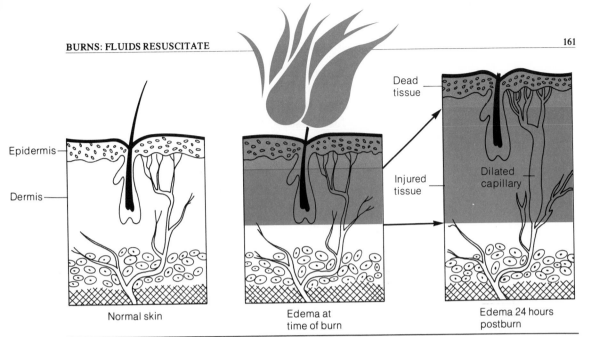

Epidermis

Dermis

Normal skin

Edema at time of burn

Dead tissue

Injured tissue

Dilated capillary

Edema 24 hours postburn

last for 2 weeks or longer. At this time parenteral fluids are changed to dextrose in water as the electrolytes in lactated Ringer's solution are no longer needed. While potassium is spilling out in the urine, it is no longer being released from the now-healing cells. So, about the 5th day, watch for and prevent hypokalemia. If untreated, hypokalemia can produce severe symptoms including weakness and muscle flaccidity; weak, irregular pulse; hypotension; anorexia and vomiting; shallow breathing; apprehension, depression or confusion.

Because the burned patient needs large amounts of potassium for cell synthesis, he needs supplements of potassium to offset this deficit, and daily electrolyte evaluations are essential to plan replacement, which may demand from 80 to 200 mEq/day. Such supplements do not usually cause hyperkalemia in the patient with adequately functioning kidneys. However, take care to keep potassium levels within normal limits if the patient is on digitalis.

Although serum *magnesium* levels may remain within low normal limits, total body magnesium may be decreased. A common sign of this problem is a total body tremor that is particularly noticeable in the extremities. Parenteral magnesium sulfate or magnesium containing antacids are often given to prevent magnesium deficit. Serum calcium levels tend to be slightly below normal but do not usually require calcium replacement.

Where edema forms

Deep partial- and full-thickness burns destroy all function in the epidermis. Beneath that layer, fluid escapes from dilated capillaries into damaged tissue causing edema. These drawings show you a crosssection of normal skin, skin at the time of injury, and skin 24 hours after the burn.

Burned skin may not expand with edema. Then, edema compresses the underlying vessels. For example, such edema of the neck and chest endangers the airway and respiratory function. Decompression escharotomy is then indicated.

Also, watch serum *chloride* concentration carefully during fluid resuscitation. Chloride is almost totally reabsorbed from the urine of burned patients; and, most I.V. solutions contain chloride. So unless fluids are switched to water when diuresis begins, the burned patient may easily become hyperchloremic. Hyperchloremia aggravates metabolic acidosis (which in trauma patients results from the release of fixed acids from injured cells and the production of lactic acid from poorly perfused tissue) by replacing some bicarbonate with chloride ions, thus diluting the buffer base. However, hypochloremia is usually a problem only when there are large amounts of nasogastric drainage.

When is resuscitation adequate? Nurses can usually consider fluid resuscitation adequate when the patient shows:
- urine volume of 30 to 60 ml/hour in adults; correspondingly less (10 to 30 ml/hr) for children, the elderly, and those with cardiac, pulmonary, or renal problems
- lucid state
- central venous pressure under 10
- pulse below 110 beats/minute; respiration below 24
- acidosis of burn shock corrected in 18 to 24 hours.

Children and the Aged
FLUID PROBLEMS DOMINATE

20

BY JOYCE KEE, RN, BSN, MSN
AND ANN P. GREGORY, RN, BSN, MSN

DO YOU KNOW HOW fluid requirements are special in children? Can you accurately assess imbalances? Start by remembering the trite but true saying, "Children are not small adults." Their body water content, compartmental proportions of fluid, and homeostatic controls are different. So are their extracellular and intracellular fluid compartments. That means their maintenance requirements for water and electrolytes are different as well.

Dehydration, a threat

Despite his generous fluid content, the younger the infant, the smaller his fluid reserve. This small reserve means great vulnerability to water deficit. Moreover, he needs a proportionately larger fluid intake and output, for several reasons: great body surface in proportion to mass (still greater in premature infants); increased metabolic rate; and immature kidneys, which require proportionately more water to excrete metabolic waste. A child's life depends on rapid turnover of water. Adults require 30 to 40 ml/kg of water every 24 hours, but a month-old infant needs 100 ml/kg. Later, he needs 50 to 70 ml/kg, depending on age, weight, and surface area.

Fluids critical in surgery

Surgery risks increase in babies and children depleted of water, sodium, and potassium, or in those with acid-base disorders. So *before surgery:*

• Assess and correct any fluid imbalance.

• Take vital signs for baseline.

• Determine electrolyte levels.

• Rapid breathing and perspiration intensify insensible water loss. Use a mist tent to minimize it. Some authorities recommend increasing fluid replacement by 10% for each 1°F. rise in temperature.

• If urinary output or kidney function is poor, establish flow with a hypotonic or isotonic infusion. With diarrhea or vomiting, determine the fluid and electrolyte replacement required. If the baby is dehydrated, start with a hypotonic saline, then use an isotonic 5% dextrose in water followed by ⅓ normal saline. Use a hypotonic solution for infants since their kidneys can't concentrate urine well. After you establish urinary flow, use a multiple electrolyte solution.

• If a child is to receive nothing by mouth before surgery, don't withhold liquids longer than 4 to 6 hours. For the hours remaining before surgery, give I.V. infusions. Then, watch for overhydration. *During surgery:*

Use glucose solutions to replace fluid loss. Don't use multiple electrolytes unless the patient's blood values and symptoms show a clear need. *After surgery:*

Immediately withhold multiple electrolytes, especially in older children, in favor of glucose or glucose with saline. Stress and trauma at this time sharply reduce water output. Postoperative hemorrhage, sweating, or hyperventilation can produce or aggravate dehydration. If gastric suction is used, replace the fluid it

Adults have a wide margin for error of fluid administration. Adults' kidneys, if healthy, will compensate for miscalculations in both diet and therapy. But, the less efficient tubules of a young baby won't.

Acidosis and electrolytes

In the newborn, the normal range of electrolytes is quite wide. At birth, hydrogen, potassium, chloride, and sodium levels are high; bicarbonate levels are low. The newborn tends to be acidotic because his metabolic rate is high, and so is his concentration of acid metabolites; and his hydrogen ion excretion is low. Within a week, or soon after birth, the serum electrolyte concentrations come closer to those of adults. But in a premature infant, or one of low birth-weight, abnormal electrolyte concentrations may continue for several weeks.

Early changes in blood chemistry due to congenital anomalies are something else again. These require special attention to his electrolyte levels and acid-base balance.

Though *potassium* levels are elevated at birth, potassium is not conserved well in infants and small children (as in elderly). When giving supplemental potassium, assess kidney function (urine output) carefully since potassium is excreted by the kidneys and hyperkalemia can cause cardiac arrest. In infants, serum potassium levels usually exceed 10 mEq/L before cardiac arrest occurs. This is not true in older children or young adults, in whom cardiac arrest occurs at levels of 8 to 9 mEq/L.

At birth, an infant's *calcium* level exceeds the mother's. Soon after birth, the infant's calcium decreases and, in low birth-weight infants, can remain low for some time. Infants do not have calcium stores in the bone as do adults.

Watch for change

Be alert for any sign of change, especially in children who have diarrhea, vomiting, pyloric stenosis, excessive sweating from fever, diabetes (in the older child), or a cardiac anomaly. Check these points:

History. The mother may be full of anxiety and not respond thoughtfully to your questions at first. So keep asking until you get a helpful response. Without implying that her actions were inappropriate, ask her what food, fluids, or home remedies she gave the child. Ask about changes in behavior and appearance. Is the child irritable? Unusually quiet? Lethargic? Does he make purposeless movements? Refuse to eat? Is there a different note in his cry?

Neurologic signs. Look for smooth-muscle irritability — a sign of potassium deficit. Is the child's abdomen distended? Is there weakness or paralysis? Are his reflexes diminished? If you see muscle twitching, it could be from calcium or magnesium deficiency but could be mistaken for a seizure. Children readily go into calcium deficiency because growing bones do not easily relinquish calcium to recirculation.

Tissue turgor. Is the child's skin a little loose? Palpate his abdomen and medial aspect of his thighs. If he is obese, his skin may seem deceptively normal. Or, if he is undernourished, that alone can cause poor tissue turgor. Otherwise, as you would in adults, look for weight loss, sunken eyes, absence of tearing and salivation, and dry mucous membranes. Look inside his mouth: A dry tongue may merely indicate mouth breathing (although some medications and vitamin deficiencies produce the same effect). With weight loss from dehydration of about 10%, the eyeballs can recede and, during infancy, the anterior fontanel may be depressed. You may not always be able to find out the child's weight before illness. But if you can, compare it with his present weight to estimate dehydration: *mild,* 2 to 4% weight loss; *moderate,* 5 to 9% loss; and *severe,* over 10% loss.

Temperature can be either low or elevated. A subnormal temperature may come from a reduced energy output. Fever increases insensible water loss. Remember that despite fever, dehydrated children's extremities may be cold because hypovolemia impedes good peripheral blood flow.

Respiration. Note the rate, depth, and pattern of his breathing. Is there hyperpnea or Kussmaul breathing? They suggest metabolic acidosis from poor hydrogen ion excretion from immature kidneys. Or the acidosis could be due to diarrhea, salicylate poisoning, or maternal diabetes mellitus. If an older child has shallow and irregular breathing, suspect metabolic alkalosis. (But this is not a reliable sign in infants, who naturally breathe irregularly.)

Thirst is hard to identify in a baby, especially one who's nauseated or has been vomiting. Actually, absence of tearing and of salivation are better clues for determining fluid deficit.

Blood pressure is not the best clue to fluid loss in children.

removes volume for volume. We often use 5% dextrose in ½ normal saline, with 1 mEq/L of potassium added for every 100 ml of gastric juice removed.

Know how to treat the three kinds of dehydration:

• Isotonic or simple (proportional water and salt loss). This is the most common kind and the easiest to treat with rapid fluid replacement. Calculate the loss over 24 hours and in severe cases replace half in the first 8 hours and half over the next 16 hours.

• Hypertonic (hypernatremia: more water lost than salt). This results from water loss through liquid stools, from low water or high solute intake, rapid breathing, poor renal function, or any combination of these.

Raise fluid volume but watch for water intoxication and convulsions from serum sodium lower than 100 mEq/L and low calcium levels. *Don't attempt rapid full correction!* Gradually reduce the excess sodium over at least 24 hours. Use 5% dextrose in water or a physiological salt diluted ¼ or ⅓. Calcium gluconate may be added to prevent tetany, twitchings, convulsions, and cardiac arrhythmias. Later, when urinary flow returns to normal, about 3 mEq/kg of potassium may be added.

• Hypotonic (hyponatremia: more salt lost than water). This imbalance can result from copious water intake, electrolyte-free fluid infusions, or excessive sweating. Low sodium levels impair cardiac and renal functions and may produce cerebral edema with seizures.

Again, *don't attempt rapid full correction.* Restrict fluid intake or give saline slowly and carefully. Too rapid correction can cause congestive heart failure and pulmonary edema, especially in a child with cardiac problems.

IN THE ELDERLY...PHYSIOLOGIC FAILURES LEAD TO IMBALANCE

Assessing elderly patients challenges your skill. Learn to distinguish between the normal signs of aging and the more severe signs of fluid imbalance. Watch for loose skin, dry cracked lips, sunken eyes, and hollow cheeks. Don't rely on generalizations. Know what is normal for your patient.

The chief vulnerabilities of the aged are fluid imbalance, electrolyte imbalance, and acidosis or alkalosis. When the body is no longer sturdy, the respiratory, renal, cardiac, and gastrointestinal systems undergo physiologic changes that affect function and fluid balance. The following patients show typical physiologic failures.

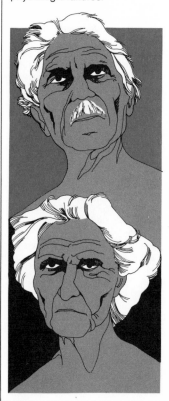

● *Respiratory.* Mrs. Cramer, 92, shows the respiratory failure so characteristic of the aged. She recently had a bout with infectious bronchitis. Partly because of that infection, but particularly because of her age, her maximal breathing capacity is greatly reduced. Her parenchymal lung tissue has lost much of its elasticity, and so has her chest wall.

Because of defective alveolar ventilation and accumulated bronchial secretions — despite medication with Isuprel and occasional use of oxygen — Mrs. Cramer's lungs inadequately diffuse respiratory gases. The reduced ventilation has increased CO_2 retention. Although there is some compensation in the rising blood bicarbonate levels, Mrs. Cramer is close to respiratory acidosis. Yet the only visible sign is shallow breathing.

Not surprisingly, Mrs. Cramer is also somewhat dehydrated. She has a low fever and a slightly rapid pulse. Not only is Mrs. Cramer coughing some fluid away, she is drinking less fluid than she needs, because her sense of thirst is less sharp, and because drinking or eating makes her chest feel congested.

● *Renal.* Mr. Brown, 79, has some generalized atherosclerosis. His parenchymal cells can no longer retain water. His urine is copious and dilute. However, if he develops renal vasoconstriction, the ischemic part of his kidney will secrete large quantities of renin and excrete less than normal amounts of water and salt.

● *Cardiac.* Mrs. Armstrong, 83, shows generalized edema. Her blood pressure is high because of increasing rigidity of the arterial walls. From pumping against resistance, and from advanced

age, her heart contractions weaken, cardiac output diminishes, stasis occurs at times throughout the circulation, and congestive heart failure increases. Blood dammed up in the venous system raises capillary pressure and forces more fluid into the tissue spaces, producing edema.

● *Gastrointestinal.* Mr. Perry, 76, suffers atrophy of the gastric mucosa common to the aging, with resulting decrease in gastric secretion, particularly of hydrochloric acid. He is subject to atrophic gastritis. A lifelong victim of the laxative habit, he has muscular atrophy in the small and large intestine, reduced motility of the gastrointestinal tract, a lessened sense of the need to eliminate, and consequent chronic constipation.

Expect dehydration

Common in the elderly, dehydration can result from increased urinary output when the kidneys can no longer concentrate urine. Excessive urine·output can also come from diminished response to ADH. Nevertheless, many elderly persons can maintain normal fluid balance — *if* they take in enough fluids. But they often do not, because:

● They have a lifelong habit of drinking very little fluid.

● They may deliberately restrict fluid intake to compensate for incontinence (especially women).

● Their physical condition may prevent them from obtaining fluids as often as they want.

● Their thirst mechanism may be blunted or absent.

Clearly, nurses need to pay particular attention to the fluid intake of elderly patients, particularly of those patients who live alone.

Tube-feeding disrupts fluids

Know and anticipate the problems of fluid imbalance likely to develop in patients who are tube-fed, as the debilitated aged so frequently are. Know what is being fed. If the feeding is high in protein (100 to 190 g), give sufficient water to help excrete the by-products of protein metabolism, and to prevent dehydration. Also be sure to consider the risk of diarrhea with tube feedings. If the feeding is spoiled, over-rich, or infused too rapidly, nausea and diarrhea will result. Check drip rate frequently. Tube feedings should generally contain no more than 150 g/day of carbohydrates; 120 g/day protein; and 120 g/day fat.

When giving tube feedings with a nasogastric or gastrostomy tube, inject 10 ml of air and listen with the stethoscope at the left side of the abdomen below the diaphragm for "popping" sounds. They'll tell you if the tube is correctly placed. Also, aspirate gastric secretions to be sure there's no retention of fluids or previous tube feedings. However, if you aspirate only gastric juices, be sure to force these back down the tube to prevent loss of needed hydrochloric acid and digestive enzymes.

Control edema

In the aged, overloading the vascular system with fluids can result in congestive heart failure and pulmonary edema. To rule out stasis edema in ambulatory patients, look for swelling of the legs in the morning, before the patient gets up and sits in a chair. Also look for dependent edema and distended neck veins. Remember that edema also causes skin and tissue breakdown, so prevent decubiti.

To control edema in patients such as Mrs. Armstrong, understand the use of digitalis and diuretics. Remember that most diuretics (except spironolactone and triamterene) make the patient excrete potassium. Laxatives and enemas also cause potassium losses. Watch the serum potassium levels carefully, and be familiar with all the signs and symptoms of potassium imbalance (see Chapter 8).

Many patients who receive diuretics need nothing more than a diet rich in potassium. The usual daily intake of potassium is 3 to 4 g. Plant foods are the principal source.

Most of all, stress the importance of physical activity. Encourage ambulatory elderly patients to move around as much as possible. Activity prevents stasis of fluid and the cellular breakdown that leads to loss of potassium and build-up of acid metabolites.

Watch for water intoxication

In the aged, water intoxication is likely to develop if they are given intravenous fluids of a hypotonic solution or an isotonic 5% dextrose in water, as well as plentiful water to drink. Because osmosis takes lesser concentration into the greater, the hypotonic vascular fluid will be drawn into the isotonic cellular area and the cells will swell.

So, always watch for symptoms of water overload in patients receiving parenteral fluids. To correct it when it happens:
- Change the I.V. fluid from a low-sodium or no-sodium solution to isotonic dextrose-saline solution or even 0.9% saline, as ordered.
- Limit water.
- Check serum sodium levels (less than 130 mEq/L).
- Notify doctor if condition persists.

Correct constipation

Constipation results from atony and atrophic changes in the lower intestines, lessened sensory awareness, and inadequate fluid intake. To correct constipation, encourage an increase in fluid intake, a more bulky diet, regular exercise, and regularity of habit. If laxatives are necessary, offer stool softeners and mild laxatives, such as milk of magnesia. Remember, however, that milk of magnesia can cause alkalosis if taken too often.

Some patients may need enemas. But remember that not all enema solutions are safe for debilitated elderly persons. For example, the often used Fleet enema contains hypertonic solution of sodium biphosphate (16 g) and sodium phosphate (6 g) — per 100 ml. If used frequently, this solution could cause dehydration by pulling water from the tissues and vascular system into the colon. Moreover, repeated enemas aggravate loss of potassium, sodium, and bicarbonate that plentifully reside in the colon. Such loss could throw a patient into electrolyte imbalance and acidosis.

Prevent diaphoresis

Ordinarily, excessive perspiration is not a common problem in the aged. However, a high room temperature or a fever can increase sweating and lead to dehydration. Correct sweating by finding and correcting the cause. Lower the room temperature if you can. If the cause is fever, offer fluids and antipyretics.

Maintaining fluid balance is essential to the precarious health of the aged. So, knowing how to evaluate and correct fluid imbalance is essential to quality health care.

I.V. anxiety

Helping hospitalized children cope with I.V. therapy requires your patience and understanding. I.V therapy usually starts early in the treatment period and ends late, and it hurts. Very young children may have to face the fright and discomfort of being restrained, often in unaccustomed positions. An uncomfortable child becomes irritable and easy to avoid.

How well the child copes depends on
- How old he is
- What coping mechanisms he's developed in the past
- What past experience he's had with medical care
- How those around him react
- Whether he associates the treatment with punishment.

You can help by encouraging the child to express his feelings and by showing him you understand. Not all children express their feelings readily, so take time to develop the child's trust. Let him handle the I.V. equipment and use it on a doll as you explain why it's necessary.

Help the child's parents cope, too. They need your explanations and support to overcome any fears, guilt feelings, or hostility they may have. Their recurring questions may mask deeper concerns you can help them express. Involve them as much as possible in the child's care so they can face the stress of this time together as a family.

The elasticity of young blood vessels tends to keep blood pressure stable. However, once the fluid volume deficit becomes severe, if it is not treated, severe shock will follow cardiovascular collapse.

Urine output. Measure the child's urine output, his stools, and his vomitus. A baby in severe fluid deficit may go 16 to 24 hours without voiding even if distended. When output decreases sharply, urine will be very concentrated as measured by specific gravity. If, despite a known fluid volume deficit, a child voids large quantities of diluted urine, it likely spells kidney damage or diabetes insipidus. The normal range of urinary output for a child: 6 months, 12 ml/hr; 1 year, 22 ml/hr; 5 years, 28 ml/hr; and 12 years, 33 to 35 ml/hr.

Stools and vomitus. Note the quantity and character of the child's stool even if it's normal. If liquid, weigh the diaper (when it belongs to a very small infant or one severely dehydrated), or estimate the loss. Record the number of times the child vomited, and the quantity and character. Bile vomitus is alkaline and calls for base fluid replacement.

Blood chemistry studies. One set of studies, showing no trends, is insufficient for assessment. Monitor hematocrit, blood electrolytes, blood urea nitrogen (BUN), and CO_2 every 4 to 8 hours, depending on severity of the fluid volume deficit. Also draw baseline arterial blood gas studies — PCO_2, pH, PO_2, and HCO_3^- — to help evaluate acid-base status and, if there are any signs of tetany, monitor calcium.

In dehydration, the hematocrit will be high. Serum sodium could be elevated, normal, or low. Serum potassium could be high or low. Upon replacement, it could either rise to normal or, as potassium is driven back into the cells where it belongs, blood levels may actually fall. If they've been elevated by fluid loss, BUN and creatinine levels should fall to normal within 48 hours after fluid replacement begins. Otherwise, suspect concomitant kidney damage. Reassess every 4 to 8 hours. In children, a deficit or overload can come very rapidly.

Diarrhea and dehydration. Diarrhea can cause three kinds of dehydration: isotonic, hypertonic, or hypotonic. To tell them apart, you need to know the history of onset, do a physical examination, and know when decreased fluid intake and diarrhea began; the number, quantity, and character of stools; and any other fluid losses. Knowing the kind of dehydration determines the choice of fluid replacement (see p. 165).

SKILLCHECK 4

1. At morning report, the night nurse tells you that Mrs. Cramer, a 92-year-old woman with acute bronchitis complicating chronic obstructive lung disease, was restless during the night and was sedated with Valium 5 mg p.o. at 2 a.m. Upon morning rounds, you find Mrs. Cramer groggy, confused, and disoriented to time, place, and person. What would you suspect the problem to be? What would you do?

2. Mr. Dwayne Marlin, a 46-year-old patient with hypertension and chronic renal failure came to the hospital twice a week for dialysis. The nursing staff knew him well since he had to be admitted every couple of months for treatment of pleural effusions. At this admission, he had a pericardial effusion. To rest his fistula, a catheter was inserted in the femoral vein for daily hemodialysis. An I.V. of normal saline with heparin was ordered to keep the lines open between treatments. This I.V. fluid was to be included in his 500 ml daily fluid allowance. Several hours after returning to the floor following his dialysis, Mr. Marlin questioned the nurses about his I.V. rate. Remembering him as a chronic worrier, the staff merely assured him that his I.V. was infusing correctly. During the evening shift, Mr. Marlin became restless and started complaining of being short of breath. Checking his vital signs, the nurse noted borderline sinus tachycardia and a slight increase in respiration, which she attributed to anxiety. By 4:00 a.m., Mr. Marlin was extremely anxious, very short of breath, with a pulse rate of 120 which was slightly irregular. What went wrong?

3. Mr. Robinson was admitted to the medical ICU with acute pulmonary edema from aortic valvular heart dis-ease. His 3-day stay in the ICU was uncomplicated, and he's now being transferred to you. His vital signs are stable at 130/90, 92, and 28. On your initial assessment you notice 3+ pitting edema of the ankles and moderate neck-vein distention at 45°. His lungs are clear to auscultation. What is causing his edema and neck-vein distention?

4. Robert Reed, a 59-year-old attorney, was brought to the E.D. by the rescue squad. He's difficult to arouse and has some cyanosis around his lips and nail beds. His BP is 180/88; pulse, 140; and respirations, 48. His arterial blood gases are pH, 7.28; PCO_2, 60 mmHg; and PO_2, 60 mmHg; and HCO_3, 38 mEq/L. What do you suppose is causing his obtunded state?

5. Mrs. Lattimer, a 50-year-old woman, is transferred to your unit from the intensive care unit where she was treated for acute pulmonary edema which resulted from decompensated hypertensive heart disease. She is presently being treated with furosemide (Lasix) 40 mg/day, and methyldopa (Aldomet) 250 mg p.o. q.i.d. She is on daily weights and has gained 2 pounds over the past 2 days. You notice she's mildly short of breath and has neck-vein distention, even though her bed is elevated to 45°. What do you suspect is happening?

6. Mrs. Sarah Williams is a 64-year-old patient with chronic renal failure. Her nursing care includes monitoring of intake and output, daily body weight, and daily electrolytes, BUN, and creatinine. You notice that Mrs. Williams' urine output has been high, ranging from 2 to 3 liters/day. Yet her BUN and creatinine are elevated. What does this mean?

(Answers on page 199)

APPLYING CORRECTIVE TECHNIQUES

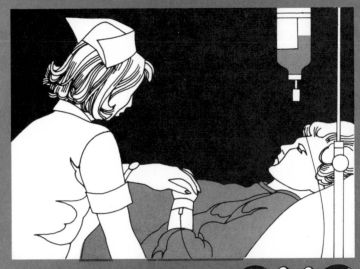

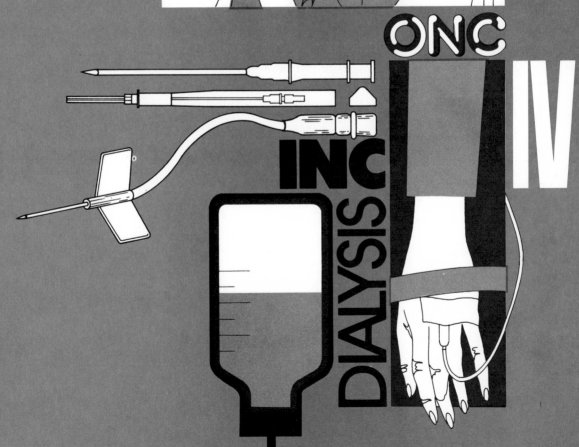

ONC

INC

IV

DIALYSIS

I.V. Therapy
TECHNIQUES TO REVIEW

21

BY CATHERINE CIAVERELLI MANZI, RN

IT'S A BUSY DAY on your unit, and you're told to start an I.V. on a patient. Do you know the four best ways to dilate a vein before placing an I.V.? The types of intracaths, when to use them and how? The nursing care involved and precautions? How the Chevron taping method differs from the "H" method? The three essential tests for infiltration? Whether you're an old hand at I.V.s or new to them, this chapter and photostory may help clear up some questions you have about them.

Preliminary checks first

Despite the importance of proper insertion, maintenance, and removal in I.V. therapy, nothing outweighs the importance of the preliminary checks you must make. Because if you fail to make them, the patient could suffer a seriously adverse reaction to the I.V., even if you give him the best technical care.

Before starting an I.V., always make sure you check the doctor's orders against the I.V. bottle from the pharmacy. Does it contain the correct fluid? Is the amount correct? Do you have all the additives ordered by the doctor? If additives are used, note and label their names, dose, rate of administra-

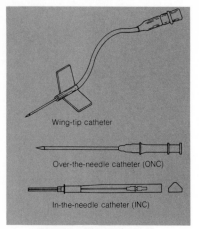

Wing-tip catheter

Over-the-needle catheter (ONC)

In-the-needle catheter (INC)

Common infusion sets
Wing-tip or *butterfly* sets
consist of a wing-tip needle
with a metal cannula, plastic or
rubber wings and a plastic
catheter and hub. The needle is ½
to 1¼ inches long. The catheter
length varies from 3 to 12 inches.
This infusion set is available in
needle gauges from 16 to 26.

The *over-the-needle catheter* is
available in gauges 12 to 22. The
needle bevel should extend
beyond the catheter, which is 1¼
to 8 inches in length.

The *in-the-needle catheter*
comes in gauges 14 to 19. The
needle length is 1½ to 2 inches
and the catheter length is 8 to 36
inches. The set also consists of a
catheter guard sleeve to keep the
catheter sterile. Once the catheter
is inserted, the bevel needle
cover is placed over the needle
and catheter to prevent severing
the catheter after it and the needle
are taped.

tion, expiration date and time on the I.V. bottle.

If the patient will be receiving several different I.V. fluids during the day, also check the solution bottle to make sure you're giving the right fluid in the right sequence.

Next, check the patient to determine the best type of equipment and the best insertion site. Will the I.V. be short-term? If so, you may use a wing-tip needle. Will it be long-term? If so, you'll probably prefer an indwelling catheter, such as an intracath or an angiocath.

Ideally, you should insert an I.V. at the distal end of a vein. But, if the patient has had numerous I.V.s, or has bruises there, you'll have to select another site — either further up the vein or in another extremity.

Stay away from areas where flexion or movement of the extremity might dislodge the needle or catheter, cause a restriction of fluid flow, or worse, bring on phlebitis due to movement of the inserted catheter. Most often, nurses choose the anterior or posterior aspect of the forearm and back of the hand, especially for prolonged, continuous fluid drip. In selecting the site, keep in mind the patient's condition, his diagnosis, and his age. Infants, small children, and old people usually have small lumens. Also consider the duration and purpose of the I.V. (short- or long-term) and the condition of the veins and their resilience. Try to avoid veins that feel hard and "rolly."

The size of the needle will help you choose the insertion site. For placing an indwelling catheter, you need a slightly larger vein than for placing a metal needle, which is usually smaller. And if you'll be using a large-gauge needle (for blood transfusions), you'll need to select an even larger vein. Remember that shallow insertion of a needle into the vein is helpful particularly in elderly patients (with poor vein tone) and young children (with small lumens).

Proceed with the I.V. only after you've made all these preliminary checks. Be sure to record the time of insertion in your notes. Keep an accurate record of the amount, type, and time of all fluids given. Write on the I.V. dressing: the date, the type and gauge of the needle or catheter, and your initials. Remember, when you change the dressing, include the above and note the date of dressing change. Remember that I.V. fluids are drugs just like any other medication. Mistakes in administration or miscalculated doses of I.V. fluids can bring on the same adverse reactions. So, give I.V. fluids with care.

Know the types of infusion sets

Infusion sets...over-the-needle catheters...through-the-needle catheters. What used to be relatively simple equipment has become more complicated, with refinements each year. Though you may rely on the I.V. team for help in such matters, you need some working knowledge of your own.

Remember three categories of I.V. apparatus: (1) infusion sets, i.e. butterfly infusion sets, (2) over-the-needle catheters (ONC); and (3) in-the-needle catheters (INC). While each differs in design, the three share at least these elements: the needle itself, which varies in gauge and size; the catheter and infusion tube, which also varies in gauge and size according to application; the luer adapter or plug; and the needle guard.

The butterfly infusion set has the advantage of a one-piece apparatus: The infusion needle and clear vinyl tubing are permanently bonded into a single unit. Another advantage is its short beveled needle, which reduces the risk of secondary puncture and infiltration from puncture of the posterior aspect of the vein wall. The wings are usually made of rubber or plastic. The catheter is also plastic, and the cannula is stainless steel. After insertion of the needle, the wings should lie flat against the patient's skin where they can be anchored securely in place with tape. This prevents the needle from rolling in the vein. Infusion units are recommended for use in children and the elderly whose veins are apt to be tiny or brittle.

ONC and INC intravenous sets are more specialized and, by both design and usage, more complex. Why are they used at all? They can perform some I.V. placements that the uncomplicated infusion sets can't. Vein catheterization, for example. Both ONC and INC sets are similarly constructed except for one major difference: They are design opposites. In other words, the ONC catheter encompasses the needle; the INC needle encompasses the catheter.

The ONC with its short, wide cannula (catheter) is considered essential for rapid infusion, or for situations where the longer INC apparatus is not needed. The longer, narrower INC catheter is preferred when prolonged infusion is called for, as in vein catheterization.

I.V. therapists generally prefer ONC or INC placements because they're more comfortable for the patient.

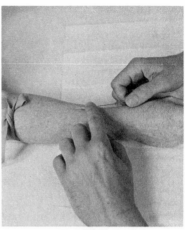

INCs and ONCs similar
Procedure is almost the same for INC and ONC placements. When placing an INC, remove the needle guard and keep it for later use. Make the venipuncture. After you see blood flashback, stop the flow by moving the luer plug into luer adapter or connector. Place the catheter into the needle sleeve or sack body and slide it forward through the needle bore and into the vein for desired length. Press on the vein just ahead of needle point to hold it during withdrawal of the needle. Grasping the needle near the hub, slide it firmly back onto adapter and open the needle guard by twisting hinged or snap closures. Then secure the needle and catheter by snapping the needle guard shut.

The one variable for ONC placement is in the catheter insertion and needle retraction phases. After venipuncture, insert the catheter through the vein by sliding the adapter along the needle until you achieve the desired limit of catheterization. Then withdraw the needle slowly while holding the catheter adapter in place.

Some Commonly Used I.V. Products

PRODUCT	ELECTROLYTES		INDICATIONS	PRECAUTIONS AND NURSING IMPLICATIONS
	ELEMENT SUPPLIED	AMOUNT SUPPLIED		
Dextrose solutions 2½% 5% 10% 50%			Maintains water balance and corrects imbalance. Supplies calories as carbohydrates	• Electrolyte-free solutions may cause peripheral circulatory collapse and anuria in patients with sodium deficiency, and may aggravate hypokalemia. Do not administer with blood
Saline solutions 0.45%	Sodium Chloride	77 mEq/L 77 mEq/L	Fluid replacement, dehydration, sodium depletion. Low salt syndrome (hyponatremia)	• Use sodium solutions with caution in edematous patients with heart, renal, or hepatic disease. Administer slowly
0.9%	Sodium Chloride	154 mEq/L 154 mEq/L		
3%	Sodium Chloride	513 mEq/L 513 mEq/L		
5%	Sodium Chloride	855 mEq/L 855 mEq/L		
Dextrose with saline 5% dextrose and 0.45% NaCl	Sodium Chloride	77 mEq/L 77 mEq/L	Fluid replacement; caloric feeding; dehydration; sodium depletion	
5% dextrose and 0.9% NaCl	Sodium Chloride	154 mEq/L 154 mEq/L		
Dextrose in Ringer's or Ringer's lactate			Replacement of surgical or GI loss; dehydration, sodium depletion, acidosis; diarrhea and burns	
Dextrose 2½%, 5%, or 10% in lactated Ringer's solution	Sodium Potassium Calcium Chloride Lactate	130 mEq/L 4 mEq/L 3 mEq/L 109 mEq/L 28 mEq/L		• Check urine flow before giving potassium

Some Commonly Used I.V. Products				
PRODUCT	ELECTROLYTES		INDICATIONS	PRECAUTIONS AND NURSING IMPLICATIONS
	ELEMENT SUPPLIED	AMOUNT SUPPLIED		
Ringer's injection (plain)	Sodium Potassium Calcium Chloride	147 mEq/L 4 mEq/L 4.5 mEq/L 155.5 mEq/L	Dehydration; sodium depletion, replacement of GI loss	
Lactated Ringer's injection U.S.P. (plain) (Hartmann's solution)	Sodium Potassium Calcium Chloride Lactate	130 mEq/L 4 mEq/L 3 mEq/L 109 mEq/L 28 mEq/L	Replacement of surgical and GI loss; dehydration; sodium depletion; acidosis; diarrhea and burns	
M/6 sodium lactate injection U.S.P. (plain)	Sodium Lactate	167 mEq/L 167 mEq/L	Severe metabolic acidosis (raises bicarbonate levels).	
5%, 10%, 20% Mannitol in 0.45% NaCl	Sodium Chloride	77 mEq/L 77 mEq/L	Test for renal function (e.g. oliguria due to tubular necrosis). Diuretic therapy for intoxications, edema,and ascites	• Do not give to patients with:impaired renal function who fail to respond to the test dose; severe CHF; metabolic edema and head injuries. Low room temperature may cause crystallization. Use blood filter set to prevent infusion of mannitol crystals
Dextran 40 10% injection with 5% dextrose 10% injection with 0.9% NaCl	Sodium Chloride	77 mEq/500 ml 77 mEq/500ml	Provides plasma volume expansion and early fluid replacement in shock when whole blood or blood products are not available or when urgency does not allow time for crossmatching	• Watch for allergic reaction such as mild urticaria. Stop infusion at first sign of reaction
Dextran 70 6% injection with 5% dextrose 6% injection with 0.9% NaCl	Sodium Chloride	77 mEq/500 ml 77 mEq/500 ml	Provides plasma volume expansion and early fluid replacement in shock and hypovolemia when whole blood or blood products are not available or when urgency does not allow time for crossmatching	• Monitor urine flow: if oliguria or anuria occurs, stop infusion. Contraindicated in dehydration or kidney disease. Do not exceed 2 grams/kg of body weight per 24 hours

Always check your equipment

Before beginning an I.V., check all equipment. Hold the I.V. bottle up to the light (Figure 1). If you see a flash of light through it, the bottle has a razor-thin crack; return it to the pharmacy. (If the solution comes in a bag, hold it up to the light and gently squeeze both sides to check for any leakage that might indicate holes.)

Always check I.V. fluids against the light for particles or discoloration. A white film or a cloudy solution indicates contamination or incompatibility of additives.

Holding the I.V. tubing up to the light, check its entire length for any discolorations (Figure 2). If you notice stains, wetness, or condensation, get a new I.V. administration set.

Next, insert the I.V. catheter

Explain the procedure to the patient and set up your equipment at his bedside.

Examine his arm and select the infusion site (Figure 3). Start an I.V. at the distal end of the vein if possible. Note the quality of blood flow, manually depress the vein, and release. Avoid veins that feel hard or like a piece of rope with hard cords or nodules above the intended site. Shave around the insertion site, making sure to remove hair where you will be applying tape.

To dilate the vein, lower his arm to below his heart and gently tap or pat the area over the vein (Figure 4). Ask him to open and close his fist. This may also help distend the veins. You may need to further dilate the vein by applying warm compresses (cover the entire length of the arm for at least 15 minutes [Figure 5]). Or apply a tourniquet for a few seconds about 6 to 8 inches above the injection site. Be sure the tourniquet isn't so tight that it will cut off arterial circulation

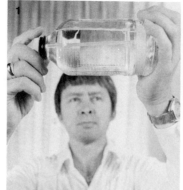

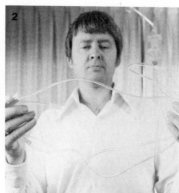

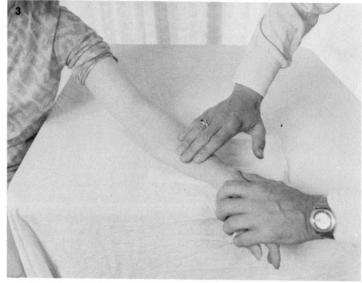

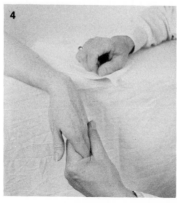

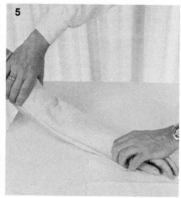

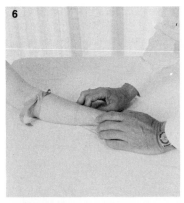

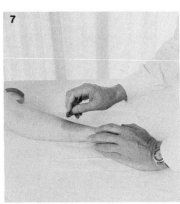

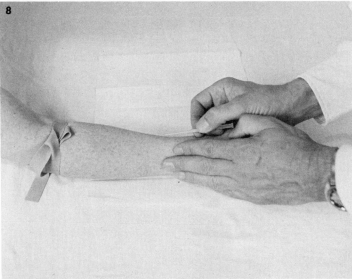

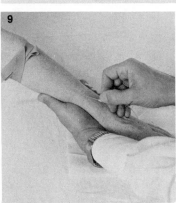

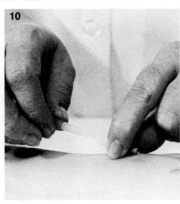

(Figure 6). If you can't feel the patient's radial pulse, the tourniquet is too tight; reapply it.

Manually apply downward distal pressure on both sides of the vein to dilate it and to prevent the patient from jerking his arm away when you insert the needle.

Cleanse the I.V. site with alcohol or another antiseptic agent.

Hold the intracath with the needle at a 45° angle along the side of the vein wall, in the direction of the insertion site (Figure 8). Pierce the skin and insert the needle into the subcutaneous tissue. Decrease the angle of the intracath until it lies parallel to the skin and slightly to one side of the vein wall.

Apply pressure with the needle in the direction of the vein and enter it. With this method, you'll run less chance of puncturing both sides of the vein, causing seepage of blood into tissues. Check for this by observing for swelling above the infusion site (Figure 9).

Remove the tourniquet and connect the I.V. tubing to the hub of the catheter. Holding the catheter securely in place, open the I.V. clamp and let the fluid run into the vein. Check to see that the solution is running freely and that there's no swelling or tenderness above the site (Figure 10).

When you hold the I.V. bottle or bag below the insertion site, gravity will cause a backflow of blood into the hub of an indwelling catheter or into the needle tubing of a wing-tip (butterfly) needle. This indicates that you're in the vein.

At any sign of infiltration, remove the catheter or needle and catheter together (if the INC type is used). Apply pressure to the insertion site and start over (with a new catheter or needle to avoid contamination).

Taping a wing-tip or butterfly needle — the Chevron method

Support the arm and place a small piece of ¼ inch tape over both wings of the needle to hold the needle in place.

Place another small piece of ¼ inch tape under the needle tubing.

Fold one end of the tape over one wing and the other end over the other wing, in crisscross fashion (Figure 1).

Coil the needle tubing in a circle over the wings, so the connector for the I.V. tubing lies just below the insertion site. Place another piece of tape over the coil, covering the first piece of tape. Place antiseptic ointment and a sterile bandage over the insertion site.

Tape the tubing again about 6 inches above the insertion site. This will prevent jiggling of the needle in the vein if someone inadvertently pulls the I.V. tubing.

The "H" Method

Place ¼ inch tape across both wings.

Apply a small piece of tape over one wing, perpendicular to the first piece of tape.

Place another piece of tape perpendicular over the other wing (Figure 2).

Coil the needle tubing in a circle over the wings so the connector for the I.V. tubing lies just below the insertion site. Apply another piece of tape across the coil, placing tape over tape (Figure 3).

As you did with the Chevron method, place antiseptic ointment and sterile bandage or Band-Aid over the insertion site; tape the connection; and make a "U" turn with the tubing and tape it below and above the insertion site.

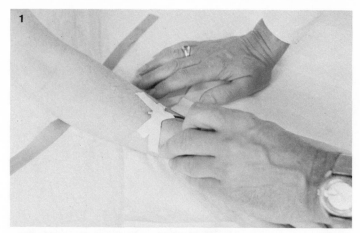

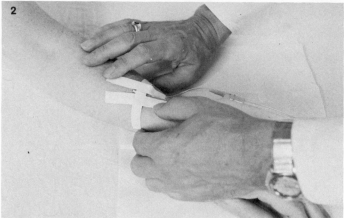

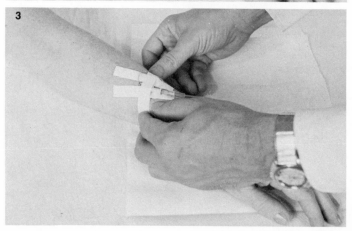

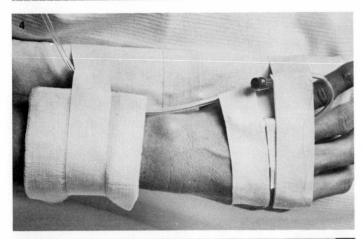

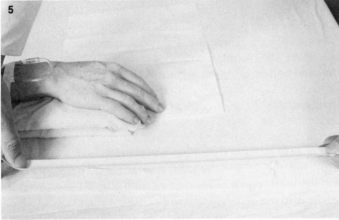

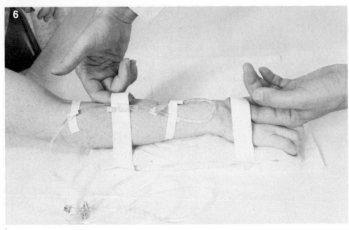

Taping an indwelling catheter

Place a small piece of tape over the hub of the catheter to secure it to the skin.

Then, place a short piece of ¼ inch tape under the I.V. tubing. Using the Chevron (crisscross) method, tape the tubing to the catheter. This will hold the catheter-tubing joint tightly together.

Apply an antiseptic ointment over the insertion site and cover it with a sterile dressing. Run the tubing down the patient's arm about 3 inches and then back up his arm, creating a "U" formation. Apply a piece of tape over both sides of the "U".

Tape the tubing again about 6 inches above the insertion site (Figure 4). This will prevent tension on the catheter at the injection site if someone inadvertently pulls the I.V. tubing.

Applying an armboard

First make sure the armboard is well padded for the patient's comfort. Place it under the patient's arm. Cut two long pieces of adhesive tape — one as long as the diameter of the patient's arm and the other twice as long. Place the adhesive sides together, making sure to center the shorter strip on the longer strip. Press together so they form a nonadhesive strip with two adhesive ends (Figure 5).

Place the nonadhesive portions of the strips over the patient's arm. Pull the adhesive ends underneath the armboard, just tight enough to leave a small space between the patient's arm and armboard (Figure 6). Fasten the adhesive ends to the armboard.

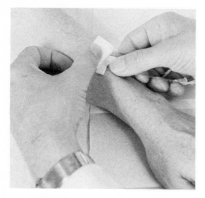

Disconnecting the I.V.
Gently remove the protective
dressing over the insertion site,
being careful not to jerk the
patient's arm.

Remove all tape. After checking
the I.V. site for any complications,
place a small dressing over the
insertion site. Using the I.V.
clamp, shut off the I.V.

Without applying any pressure,
quickly pull back on the cannula
of the catheter or needle and
remove. Don't pull up on the
cannula during removal since that
could traumatize the vein.
Immediately apply firm pressure
on the dressing over the site to
prevent a hematoma. Also hold
the patient's arm up in the air for a
couple of minutes to drain blood
away from the site.

Apply a sterile dressing or
Band-Aid over the site and leave it
in place until you check the site
later for complications.

Checking the I.V. site for complications

Always keep the insertion site covered with a sterile dressing
to help prevent airborne contamination. Periodically, lift one
side of the dressing to inspect the site for local complications.
Look for: any change in skin color around the site, which
might indicate phlebitis; any moisture or fluid around the site
(bacteria will thrive on the glucose); and, any purulent drainage, which indicates an infection. If you find any of these
conditions, immediately change the I.V. to another site.

You can check for infiltration in several ways. First, you can
check the arm for edema around the injection site; be sure to
compare both arms for size since swelling may not be noticeable otherwise. Check for edema on the posterior side of the
patient's arm, too. If the needle punctured both sides of the
vein during insertion, fluids will be infiltrating the subcutaneous tissue on the posterior side.

Also check the temperature of the skin around the insertion
site. Since I.V. solution will be about 68° F. (room temperature) and normal body temperature is 98.6° F. (37° C.), the skin
will feel cold if solution is infiltrating the subcutaneous tissue.
Finally, check for infiltration by trying to stop the flow. Apply
a tourniquet or manual pressure about 4 to 6 inches above the
insertion site. Open the I.V. clamp all the way. If the I.V.
continues to run, it is running into the subcutaneous tissue; if it
stops, the needle is in the vein. Another test — hold the I.V.
solution bottle down below the insertion site. If the catheter or
needle is in the vein, gravity will cause the backflow of blood
into the catheter and tubing.

Periodically check the flow rate to make sure no problems
exist. If the I.V. tubing is below bed level, the flow will slow or
stop because the fluid will have to run uphill and a backflow of
blood will result.

To correct the problem, coil up the excess I.V. tubing and
place a rubber band around it, loosely. Make sure that the
tubing doesn't kink from the rubber band. Using tape, attach
the rubber band to the bed. Check the tubing after the patient
changes position to make sure he isn't lying on it and that it
isn't kinked (which causes the flow rate to change). And watch
those side rails!

Hyperalimentation
A PLUS FOR NITROGEN BALANCE

22

BY RITA COLLEY, RN, BA
AND JEAN WILSON, RN, BS

TOTAL PARENTERAL NUTRITION (TPN) or hyperalimentation?
Do you know how to give it? Why patients need it? Its complications? Your nursing responsibilities?

Who needs hyperalimentation? Someone like Mrs. Jones, a
36-year-old housewife who had two operations for regional
enteritis. Postop, she developed multiple fistulas around her
abdominal wound. She was extremely anorexic, with nausea
and vomiting. When her weight dropped 60 lbs, her doctor
prescribed hyperalimentation.

If you care for patients who need TPN, you need to know
how to explain the procedure to them and their families, how
to prepare the solutions, and how to handle the equipment and
what precautions to take.

What is it?
It is the intravenous infusion of protein as amino acid (nitrogen) and hypertonic glucose and additives (including vitamins, electrolytes and minerals, and trace elements). The
nitrogen source is a crystalline amino acid solution (FreAmine,
Aminosyn, Travisol). In a patient like Mrs. Jones whose
caloric intake is insufficient and does not provide enough

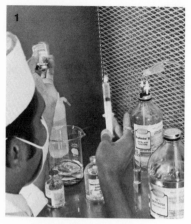

TPN procedure
The two common vessels used to insert a TPN infusion are the subclavian vein and the jugular vein. Once inserted, the catheter should terminate in the superior vena cava. Try not to use the brachial and femoral veins; they're usually contraindicated because they produce a high incidence of thrombophlebitis and limit movement of the extremities. In addition, kinking of the catheter could result.

Solutions are usually mixed aseptically in the pharmacy under a Laminar flow hood. This prevents any airborne contamination during the mixing. If the TPN solutions are to be mixed on the floor, follow the manufacturer's suggestions (Figure 1).

Check the bottle for any cracks and the solution for clarity. And double-check the time and expiration date of the solution. Make sure that the bottle label matches the doctor's order sheet. If additives (i.e., electrolytes) are to be used, maintain sterile technique: Remove the pharmacy-sealed cap, leaving the yellow latex diaphragm in place (this assures a vacuum); wipe with alcohol and inject the additives (Figure 2). Cover with an

protein-sparing calories, the body breaks down its protein and fat for energy. Excessive amounts of nitrogen are lost in the urine, and the patient goes into negative nitrogen balance. Severe weight loss, debilitation, dehydration, electrolyte imbalances, emaciation, and death may follow.

So, TPN can provide Mrs. Jones with calories, maintain positive nitrogen balance, and supply or replace needed essential vitamins, electrolytes and minerals. Therefore TPN promotes tissue synthesis, wound healing, and normal metabolic function. In certain diseases (ulcerative colitis, GI fistulas, and granulomatous colitis) TPN is used to allow the gastrointestinal tract to rest. It decreases activity of the gallbladder, pancreas, and small intestines. It often allows healing without surgery. But if surgery becomes necessary, the patient may be better able to tolerate it after TPN preparation. Patients so prepared develop fewer complications.

Patients who have had extensive bowel surgery and develop the short-gut syndrome also do well with TPN. As you know, the short-gut syndrome usually occurs after extensive resective surgery; areas within the small bowel decrease in their ability to absorb, and this leads to an obligatory nitrogen loss and imbalance and intestinal inability to handle normal nutritional needs. Temporarily nourishing the patient with TPN infusion gives the remaining small intestine time to compensate for altered physiology and eventually handle the body's nutritional and metabolic needs.

Severely burned patients, also in negative nitrogen balance, benefit from TPN, show faster wound healing and formation of granulation tissue, and sometimes respond better to skin grafting. Their rate of sepsis seems decreased, although extreme care and monitoring needs to be maintained throughout the course of TPN and hospitalization.

After TPN, Mrs. Jones' anorexia, nausea, vomiting, and abdominal pain diminished significantly. X-rays showed improvement in the appearance of her gastrointestinal tract and closure of her fistulas. She started to gain weight and surgery was postponed.

Watch for complications
Some complications that can occur in patients receiving TPN: septicemia, fungal infection, air emboli (which are catheter-related), hemothorax, hydrothorax, pneumothorax

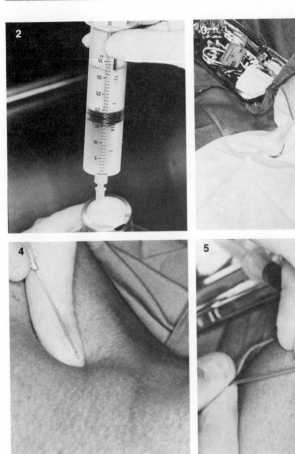

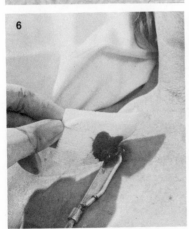

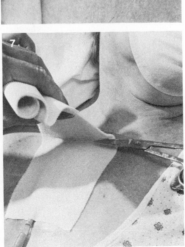

airtight cap. If solution is used immediately, remove latex diaphragm and attach I.V. tubing into outlet. Prime I.V. tubing and filter with the solution.

Placing the catheter

Place the patient in Trendelenburg's position with his head hyperextended. This allows easier vein access, increases venous pressure, and dilates the blood vessels.

Shave the site of insertion and clean it with acetone, iodine and alcohol. The doctor will then drape the patient with surgical drapes (Figure 3).

Next, he will infiltrate the area with a local anesthetic (lidocaine 1%) and insert a 14 gauge needle into the vein (Figure 4).

During the venous placement of the catheter, the catheter is open to air, so to prevent an air embolus the patient is asked to bear down with his mouth closed. This is the Valsalva maneuver. Note backflow of blood (Figure 5).

Once the catheter is inserted, it is connected to the I.V. tubing. Usually a single suture is used to secure the catheter. Multiple sutures increase the chance of inflammation and of kinking of the catheter. The doctor will place a plastic needle guard around the needle and catheter to prevent an accidental piercing of the patient's skin.

An antibacterial-antifungal ointment is applied to the catheter insertion site (Figure 6). An occlusive dressing is applied. This maintains sterility, and immobilizes and protects the catheter and needle (Figure 7). A chest X-ray should be taken immediately after, to confirm catheter tip placement and to highlight any complications. Infuse isotonic solutions only until correct catheter placement is confirmed. Infuse slowly.

Changing TPN solution and tubing

Remove the tape that secures the tubing and filter to the dressing. Aseptically attach a new adult infusion set to the bottle of solution. Prime the tubing and tap the end gently to dislodge any solution droplets (Figure 1).

Being careful not to contaminate the filter, connect the infusion set to the filter housing (Figure 2). Remove the protective covering from the distal end of the filter and discard it. Hold the filter housing below the I.V. bottle. Prime the tubing according to the manufacturer's directions.

Gently tap the housing with your finger to dispel any air trapped distal to the membrane. Tap the end to free the droplets (Figure 3). Using a clamp for leverage, quickly replace the old tubing with a new one, while the patient performs Valsalva's maneuver (Figure 4).

Readjust the flow rate. Reanchor the filter with 1-inch adhesive. Date the tubing.

Changing the TPN dressing

Gather the equipment you'll need at the patient's bedside. Explain the procedure to him. Pour out the solutions. Use aseptic technique throughout the procedure. Wear sterile gloves and a face mask. The patient should wear a face mask, too, unless contraindicated (Figure 5).

Place the patient in a supine position with his head turned laterally. Remove the old tape and dressing carefully. Wear sterile gloves if you're going to touch underneath the dressing. Put on a new pair of sterile gloves before continuing with the procedure (Figure 6).

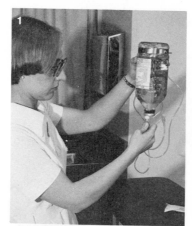

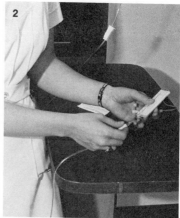

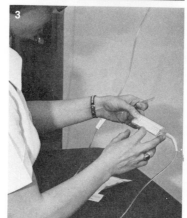

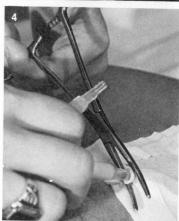

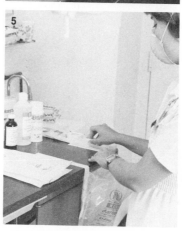

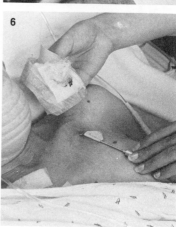

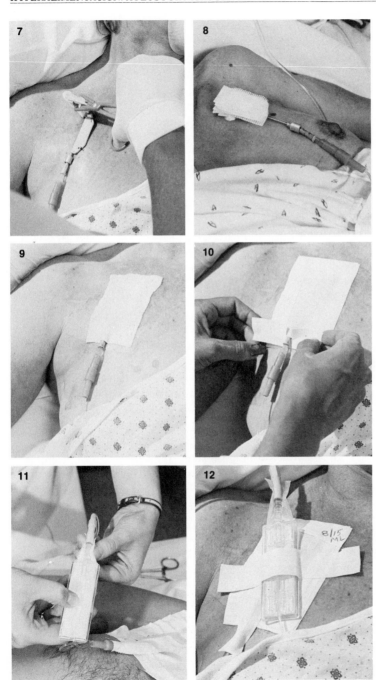

Apply a gauze sponge to the end of a sterile clamp. Start with the acetone, a defatting agent that removes dead cells. Scrub the site with the acetone, using the "clean to dirty method," that is, scrubbing in a circular fashion moving from in near the site outward. Use a gentle abrasive action, but be careful not to irritate the patient's skin. Then use iodine, an antifungal and antibacterial agent. Scrub for a full 2 minutes and then let this solution dry in the air. Finally, cleanse the skin of all iodine, using alcohol (Figure 7).

Apply Betadine ointment to the catheter site and spray the surrounding skin with tincture of benzoin to make the dressing adhere better. Place a small gauze dressing over the insertion site, leaving part of the catheter and hub exposed (Figure 8). Note: Cover ⅔ of the hub with a sterile adhesive bandage, making sure it also covers the gauze sponges. This provides for easier access to the hub during I.V. tubing changes. Secure the catheter needle to the skin by placing a sterile adhesive bandage as shown (Figure 9).

Border three edges of the dressing with tape. Make a small slit in a fourth piece of tape and place it under the hub. This guarantees an occlusive seal (Figure 10).

Secure all I.V. tubing junctions, all catheter hub junctions, and the filter with adhesive tape to protect against accidental separation (Figure 11).

To prevent traction on the catheter, anchor the filter and tubing to the dressing (Figure 12). Note the time and date of the changing on the tape and in your Notes. Remember to include the condition of the patient's skin and the date of the catheter insertion.

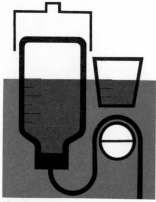

Nursing tips
- Infuse TPN solution at a constant rate. If the fluid falls behind schedule, recalculate the flow rate. *Do not catch up!* Radical shifts in fluid rate can cause metabolic problems.
- Generally patients spill +2 urine glucose during the first 2 days of TPN until their pancreas adjusts to the new glucose load.
- If TPN solution is unavailable, give 20% dextrose. Remember, infuse at the same flow rate.
- Discontinue TPN gradually, allowing the body to adjust to lower levels of glucose. Isotonic glucose solution may be administered for at least 12 hours after to protect against rebound hypoglycemia.
- Label the TPN solution bottle (date, time of expiration and hanging, rate, and any additives).
- Don't use the line for drawing or giving blood, medications, or piggy-backing other solutions.
- Patients who have a tracheostomy, problems of secretions, or a draining wound, or a high-humidity oxygen mask, need a water-proof sterile covering over the TPN site.
- Tell TPN patients that they may have fewer bowel movements.
- You can help a patient perform the Valsalva maneuver correctly by pressing down on his abdomen while the patient bears down.

and pleural effusion. A tingling sensation of the fingers, pain, or weakness in the arm may indicate brachial plexus injury and should be reported to the doctor. Acute fluid overload can lead to pulmonary edema and congestive heart failure. Observe for bibasilar rales, rapid thready pulse, shortness of breath, dyspnea, an increase or decrease in blood pressure, decreased urine output. Watch for signs and symptoms of an air embolus. This can occur while the central venous system is exposed to air during tubing change.

Signs and symptoms of air embolism are cyanosis, hypotension, a rapid and weak pulse, elevated venous pressure, loss of consciousness, and changes in the heart sounds. Immediate treatment: Place the patient on his left side in Trendelenburg position to keep the air in his right ventricle and prevent it from entering the pulmonary circuit. Air emboli can be fatal. So, make all tubing changes swiftly, while the patient performs the Valsalva maneuver while lying flat in bed.

Hyperglycemia, another complication, can occur when the amount of glucose-infused exceeds that which the body can metabolize. The only real sign is *glycosuria,* although serum glucose determinations should be done also. The causes of hyperglycemia are an *excess of hyperalimentation fluid, or an inability to tolerate glucose.* Hyperglycemia can cause osmotic diuresis and proceed to dehydration and coma, if it is severe and uncorrected. On the other hand, *hypoglycemia* results from decreased flow rate, a clogged filter, kinked catheter tubing, malfunctioning catheter, abrupt withdrawal of hypertonic glucose, or too much insulin. Its signs and symptoms: weakness, trembling, sweating, headache, chills, decreased level of consciousness, convulsions, hunger, increased vital signs, and apprehension. Watch for possible complications during TPN. Record and report them promptly. Remember that maintenance of asepsis is crucial before, during, and after the procedure.

Don't underestimate the importance of teaching patients and their families to understand the procedure. Patients have many understandable fears during TPN. They greatly fear having their heart perforated by the catheter, and never regaining their appetite. The TPN procedure itself is alarming to the patient. You can help a lot with a simple explanation, a smile, the touch of a hand, and a reassuring look. Patients on TPN need all the reassurance and emotional support they can get.

Dialysis
RENAL AND PERITONEAL

23

BY LOUISE JULIANI, BSN, MS

CARING FOR THE PATIENT in renal failure can be a real challenge. The challenge? Trying to reduce protein catabolism, prevent fluid and electrolyte imbalance, correct imbalance, if it occurs, and prevent infection.

When the accumulated products of metabolism, excess fluids and electrolytes can no longer be managed by dietary or fluid measures, some form of dialysis is needed. It may also be needed even for the transplant patient as a therapeutic supplement. Dialysis acts on the principle of a semipermeable membrane which leaves large molecules in the blood but allows smaller molecules to pass through. In this way, unwanted substances can be removed from the blood.

Hemodialysis most used

In hemodialysis, the blood gets perfused outside the body through a chamber lined with a semipermeable membrane (usually cellophane). On the other side of the membrane lies the dialyzing fluid. The artificial membrane substitutes for the nephrons; it readily allows the passage back and forth of small molecules such as urea or sodium, while mostly keeping back the large molecules such as proteins, glucose, or blood cells.

Complications of dialysis
Blood loss (from dialyzer leaks, or clotting)
Hemorrhage (from heparinization)
Hemolysis
Pyrogenic reaction
Hypotension or *hypertension*
Arrhythmias (from potassium imbalance)
Muscle cramps (from hypocalcemia)
Disturbed sensorium (dialysis disequilibrium syndrome)
Anemia, possibly with splenomegaly (may require transfusions and splenectomy)
Hepatitis (transmitted by transfusing blood, blood products, patients, or staff)
Accelerated atherogenesis (stroke and myocardial infarction are the leading causes of death in patients on dialysis for more than 5 years.)

Hemodialysis does its work by a combination of osmosis, diffusion, and filtration through the membrane, enhanced by positive pressure in the blood chamber or negative pressure in the dialyzing channels to promote bulk flow. The standard dialysis fluid is an aqueous solution containing cations found in blood — sodium, potassium, calcium, and magnesium, along with the anion, chloride, also prominent in blood, and acetate, which the body readily turns into bicarbonate. The non-electrolyte solute glucose may also be added. The original composition of the dialyzing fluid and its adjustment during use allow the metabolic products (urea, creatinine, and uric acid) to be removed from the body along with excessive potassium, sodium, magnesium, phosphate, and excess fluid.

Nurses monitor dialysis
Most patients undergoing hemodialysis are treated as outpatients in hospitals or satellite clinics. There the responsibility for their well-being while on hemodialysis most often lies with the nurse. Her responsibilities include: the patient's well-being during the treatment; care in monitoring of equipment; and teaching and psychosocial counseling of the patient and family.

Before each hemodialysis treatment, the nurse sets up the equipment and solution and obtains baseline patient data, including weight and vital signs. Under strict asepsis, she begins treatment by connecting the blood lines from the dialyzer to the appropriately positioned needles that have been placed in the arteriovenous fistula. Blood samples are drawn at this time for baseline laboratory values.

During the treatment, the nurse monitors the patient's comfort; measures blood pressure, pulse, respirations, temperature, weight, and clotting time; and watches for complications. There may be blood loss from dialyzer leaks or clotting in the tubing; heparinization may lead to hemorrhage; there may be hemolysis, pyrogenic reactions, hypotension, hypertension, arrhythmias from potassium imbalance, muscle cramps from hypocalcemia, or dialysis disequilibrium syndrome from cerebral edema. Treatment is usually done 2 to 3 times per week for a total of 8 to 18 hours. To end the treatment, blood samples are taken, the blood remaining in the machine is returned to the patient, and the needles removed from the arteriovenous fistula. Pressure is applied over the needle insertion site until bleeding stops. A pressure dressing is applied. Measurements taken at the beginning of treatment are repeated to determine effectiveness.

No less important, the nurse has a vital role in teaching the patient and his family about dietary restriction, medications, and the problems of chronic renal failure unaffected by dialysis, such as anemia or osteodystrophy; in counseling; and in referring patients to other help with the immense psychosocial problems that accompany chronic renal failure.

Peritoneal dialysis

Peritoneal dialysis is another available method — one that has been used since the 1940s to treat renal failure. It's safe, inexpensive, and nearly as effective as hemodialysis.

This technique consists of infusing a solution into the peritoneal cavity through a closed drainage system. It uses the peritoneum itself as a dialyzing membrane to replace the malfunctioning kidneys. The peritoneum's filtering surfaces — about 22,000 square centimeters — approximates the surface of the glomerular capillaries. This membrane lines the walls of the abdominal cavity with its own parietal surface and wraps the abdominal organs inside its visceral one. In peritoneal dialysis, the fluid is instilled into the peritoneal cavity between these two layers and left there for a controlled length of time.

Dwell time critical

But if the fluid is left in the peritoneal cavity too long, the *two fluids* — blood and bath — begin to approximate each other. More glucose molecules are absorbed despite their size. Further clearance of urea from the blood drops sharply. For this reason, dwell time should only be 20 to 30 minutes. This means the fluid should run in within 10 to 15 minutes, dwell for 20 to 30 minutes, and then drain 15 to 20 minutes.

Clearance of the blood in peritoneal dialysis is influenced by other factors, too, besides glucose concentration. For example, warming the dialysis fluid enhances solute clearance. Urea clearance, for example, is 35% greater at body temperature (37° C. or 98.6° F.) than at room temperature (25° C. or 77° F.). Warming the fluid also decreases discomfort and prevents the patient from losing body heat. A rapid exchange — finishing the job in an hour — also increases the efficiency of dialysis. So does volume. As compared to a liter an hour, 3

Gaining access

Several vascular access routes can deliver the patient's blood to the dialyzer. The access currently preferred is an internal arteriovenous fistula. Side-to-side, side-to-end, or end-to-end anatomoses connect the radial artery with an adjacent vein; skin then covers the fistula. Although the forearm is the most commonly used site, you can use the upper arm or leg instead. A well-constructed fistula may be used for years.

Other routes of access include external shunts, or internal fistulas constructed with autogenous saphenous vein grafts, bovine grafts, or Dacron prostheses.

How the catheter is inserted

Before the doctor arrives, gather the following equipment: disposable razor and blade, dialysis administration set, peritoneal dialysis solution (as ordered), local anesthesia (Xylocaine 1%), sterile gloves, Betadine solution and ointment, suture and needle (2-0 silk), and Elastoplast. Also get a sterile prepackaged dialysis tray with catheter, connector, syringes, needles, sterile dressings, and fine mesh gauze.

Explain the procedure to the patient and get his signed consent. Weigh him to obtain a baseline weight, and take temperature, pulse, respiration, and blood pressure readings. Have him empty his bladder to reduce the risk of bladder perforation during insertion. Make him comfortable in a supine position, and shave his abdomen from the umbilicus to 5 cm below it. The doctor will then begin the insertion procedure.

First, he swabs the skin with Betadine, to eliminate surface bacteria (Figure 1).

After draping the patient, he then infiltrates the skin and subcutaneous tissues with a local anesthetic (Figure 2).

He makes a small midline stab wound 3 to 5 cm below the umbilicus (Figure 3).

Next, he inserts the peritoneal catheter with stylet through the incision (Figure 4).

If the patient is thin, the doctor may inject 1 to 2 liters of fluid through the incision before inserting the stylet. This allows the mesentery and bowel to move freely when the stylet perforates the peritoneum.

With the stylet in place, have the

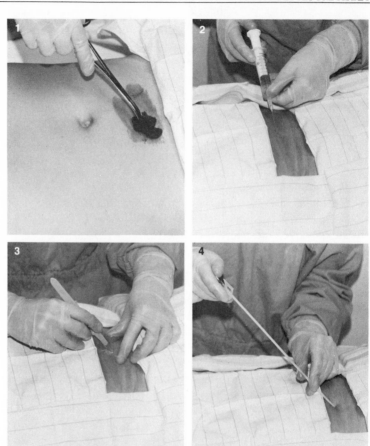

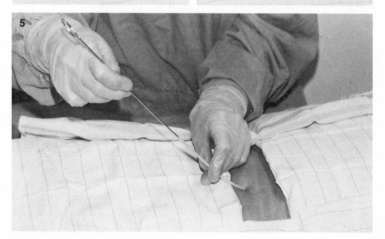

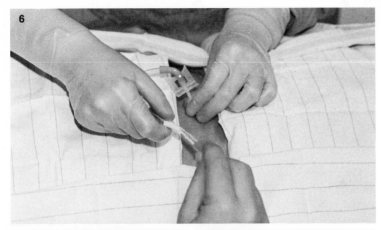

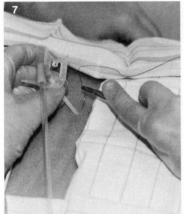

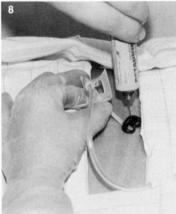

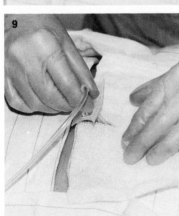

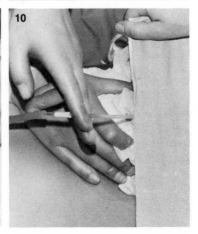

patient raise his head to tighten his abdominal muscles. This makes penetration easier and reduces the risk of injury to the intra-abdominal organs. When the doctor punctures the peritoneum, he will hear an audible pop; resistance will reduce markedly. He then removes the stylet (Figure 5).

He maneuvers the catheter into place and connects it to the administration set and dialyzing solution (Figure 6).

With a purse-string suture, he then closes the skin, looping the suture around the catheter and tying it in place (Figure 7).

He applies Betadine ointment or another antibacterial agent to the incision site (Figure 8).

Then, he places a sterile dressing around the catheter (Figure 9). After padding the area with more sterile gauze, he applies Elastoplast tape to keep the dressing and catheter in place (Figure 10).

He is then ready to allow 2 liters of warmed 37° C. dialyzing solution to run in rapidly, over a period of 10 to 15 minutes.

What to record
• Exact time of beginning and end of each infusion
• Amount infused, recovered, and any deficit or excess
• Color of outflow (clear yellow, suggests normal; cloudy, suggests infection; fecal matter suggests perforation of bowel)
• Number of exchanges
• Medication additives
• Assessment of patient's condition (vital signs; any bleeding; any leakage around catheter)
• Pre- and post-dialysis weight.

Restoring balance

How does peritoneal dialysis work? By a combination of osmosis, diffusion, and filtration, it drains off metabolic waste products and reestablishes fluid and electrolyte balance. Because the membrane is semipermeable, water and the usual solutes can pass back and forth much more freely than large protein and sugar molecules.

With peritoneal dialysis, fluid balance is attained by using bath solutions of varying tonicity or concentration. A dialyzing solution with a serum-like electrolyte content, although ordinarily without potassium, is used. If potassium is needed, you can add about 4 mEq per liter. You can also add glucose or dextrose to increase tonicity. This also increases peritoneal clearance, simply because the increased osmolarity (osmotic strength) of the higher concentrate drags more solutes out with the water.

liters will nearly double the clearance of urea. But for most adults, 2 liters an hour is the most comfortable, so this is often the standard volume exchanged.

Chronic peritoneal dialysis has become feasible since the development of special catheters that can be surgically inserted for long-term use, and of automated peritoneal dialysis equipment that does away with frequent bottle changes. The most common use of peritoneal dialysis, though, is in acute renal failure using the two-bottle system.

Care in acute peritoneal dialysis

Before any peritoneal dialysis equipment is brought to the bedside for this minor surgical procedure, the doctor should explain what is involved to the patient and his family. You should be there during the doctor's explanation so you'll know what the patient understands and expects.

Dialysis will start to solve the problem of azotemia, but it's up to you to see that the strictest sterile technique is used, and that the fluid balance and electrolytes swing toward the norm, not away from it. (For step-by-step descriptions of the procedure see photos, pp. 192-193.)

During the first exchange, take blood pressure and pulse every 15 minutes; take them every hour after that. Take the temperature every 4 hours — and *after* the abdominal catheter is removed. One of your most important jobs throughout is respiratory care. Long periods of hypoventilation enforced by a full abdomen aggravate the risk of pneumonia. Raise the head of the patient's bed, and encourage coughing and deep breathing. Turn the patient from side to side when you can. If he shows marked difficulty in breathing during dialysis, drain the fluid at once and notify the doctor. Also watch for pain, leakage of solution, bleeding, and infection.

If you must leave while your patient is being dialyzed, you must tell the person who relieves you the exact status of the exhange, and how to continue the recording. This is a common source of error. Be sure to record all the patient's intake and output (whether the latter is urine, feces, or emesis). Most important, make the patient feel that it is *he* and not the dialysis that is the focal point. Explain everything that he wants to know. Let him help when you can. And never underestimate the job you're doing. Hemo- and peritoneal dialysis need astute, intelligent, and well-organized nursing care to succeed.

SKILLCHECK 5

1. Mr. Sealy, a 66-year-old man, was admitted to your unit for cataract surgery. He needs an I.V. (5% dextrose in water) to keep his vein open. You find him obese. Even when you place a tourniquet on his arm, his veins are barely detectable. What would your next move be?

2. You've applied a tourniquet 6" to 8" above the intended site for an in-the-needle catheter by placing the patient's arm down at his side and resting on an over-bed table. You pierce his skin and enter the vein. There is no backflow of blood in the view chamber but you see a swelling proximal to the insertion site. What went wrong? What will you do next?

3. On making your I.V. rounds you discover that Mrs. Teasdale's I.V. is infusing slowly, even after you open the I.V. rate regulator all the way. Which of the following would you do about it?
   a) Discontinue the I.V. and notify the doctor.
   b) Let it go; it is a keep-open I.V.
   c) Check to see if the catheter is in the vein; by lowering the I.V. bottle below the site, apply a tourniquet 6 inches above the site or bend the I.V. tubing, distal to the site and squeeze the flashbulb. While doing one of the above, observe for a flashback of blood into the view chamber or I.V. tubing.
   d) Once the catheter in the vein is established, try pulling back on the catheter, as it may be lying against the vein wall. Check flow rate.

   e) Try elevating or depressing the catheter, by placing cotton, 2x2 guaze pad, folded 4x4 gauze pad or tongue blade under the catheter to elevate it or on top of the I.V. site and tape it down to depress the catheter. Check flow rate.

4. A patient on your unit is receiving total parenteral nutrition (TPN) during treatment for regional ileitis (Crohn's disease). Her third bottle is infusing at the ordered rate of 60 ml/hour. While making your I.V. rounds, you notice that the I.V. is infusing too slowly and is, in fact, 150 ml behind schedule. So you increase the drip rate above 60 ml/hour to compensate for lost time and get back on schedule. During the next shift, the nurse finds that this patient's fractional urine is 4⁺ for sugar. In looking over the patient's fractional urine record, she finds that this is the first time she has spilled sugar. Her serum glucose that same morning was normal. What went wrong? How could this glycosuria have been prevented?

5. Which patient situation listed below is a likely indication for TPN? Ulcerative colitis with diarrhea and weight loss? Premature infant with diarrhea and congenital gastrointestinal abnormalities? Postoperative bowel surgery? Preoperative patients with fistulas or open draining abdominal wounds after fistula repair and 10% weight loss or more? Or patients with severe burns?

(Answers on page 199)

SKILLCHECK ANSWERS

ANSWERS TO SKILLCHECK 1 (page 39)

Situation 1 — Sarah Friedman
Syndrome of inappropriate antidiuretic hormone (SIADH) is a strong possibility. Oat-cell tumors can secrete a hormone that cannot be distinguished from ADH. Mrs. Friedman's positive water balance (intake > output), low serum sodium, low urine output, and sudden weight gain strongly suggest inappropriate ADH secretion.

Patients with inappropriate ADH secretion also show serum osmolality below 280 mOsm/kg and may also have neurological symptoms including restlessness, convulsions, and unresponsiveness. Inappropriate ADH secretion is also a potential problem in patients with central nervous system disorders (such as cerebrovascular accident), hypothyroidism, and certain organic intracranial diseases.

Situation 2
The extracellular, made up of interstitial and vascular compartments, is more vulnerable to fluid loss. The intracellular compartment is generally the last to be influenced by disease states that cause changes in body fluid.

Situation 3
It may impair his sense of thirst, and so his fluid intake may be less than he needs for normal metabolism.

Secondary causes of dehydration in the elderly include increased urinary output (because kidneys can no longer concentrate urine) and diminished response to ADH (which causes an excessive amount of water to be excreted with solutes).

Situation 4 — Jerry Miller
Chronic cirrhosis impairs the synthesis of albumin by the liver. Impaired synthesis of albumin causes a decrease in his plasma colloidal osmotic pressure. Without this pressure from the plasma proteins, there's nothing to balance the hydrostatic pressure within the capillaries. This permits an excess of fluid to leave the intravascular compartment and collect in the interstitial spaces. In Mr. Miller, fluid accumulated in the peritoneal cavity, producing ascites.

Situation 5
False. Fluid intake also includes oxidative water resulting from the metabolism of food.

A certain amount of water intake is accounted for by the amount of water formed in metabolism through the oxidation of hydrogen in food or of the body tissues themselves. Water is also formed in the tissues through polymerization (synthesis) of various compounds (the reverse of hydrolysis). An ordinary mixed diet yields from 300 to 350 g of oxidative water daily. When no food or drink is taken, the body materials themselves (glycogen, protein, and fat), are used for this purpose.

Situation 6
Density of urine is another way of saying specific gravity. The specific gravity of urine (normally from 1.003 to 1.030) measures the quantity of dissolved solids present in the urine and reflects the kidneys' concentrating ability.

Situation 7
An infant's higher metabolic rate requires more water expenditure; and, the infant's immature kidneys have a lesser ability to concentrate urine, so they use more water — roughly twice as much — during normal excretion.

Situation 8 — Mr. George
Lasix would *not* only fail to relieve his symptoms but would probably throw him into alkalosis. Lasix would diurese Mr. George but also cause him to lose potassium. He had already been losing potassium through nasogastric suctioning. Without adequate replacement, he could easily become alkalotic. In patients with hepatic disease who become alkalotic, the kidneys divert ammonia from excretion in the urine to the generalized circulation and thus intensify the signs and symptoms of hepatic encephalopathy. Notice another important symptom — nausea — along with decreased urinary output. Presence of hepatic disease plus intense hypotension due to hemorrhagic shock may have caused renal damage. Mr. George's edema may have been due to this instead of liver disease. So, closer monitoring of renal function with urine specific gravities, urine sodiums, and BUN and

creatinine would help to determine if renal function is impaired. Lab tests showed that Mr. George was not in renal failure. Considering all these factors, the doctors did not prescribe Lasix. Instead, he ordered I.V. infusions of salt-poor albumin along with potassium replacement to reduce edema and ascites and to correct potassium depletion.

Situation 9

All but one of these factors (the exception: alcohol) promote retention of sodium and water by increasing the secretion of antidiuretic hormone (ADH).

ANSWERS TO SKILLCHECK 2 (page 75)

Situation 1 — Eric Winter

The first priority is fluid replacement to combat obvious hypovolemia. He will need volume expanders to maintain renal output, so careful monitoring of intake and output is extremely important. The scheduled surgery to remove obstruction will aggravate the loss of extracellular fluid into interstitial tissues, compounding the hypovolemia. If fluid replacement is adequate (infusions of albumin and appropriate crystalloid solutions with electrolytes, as needed), the fluid trapped in the bowel will be reabsorbed when healing begins. At this point, he will need special monitoring for fluid overload and subsequent congestive heart failure or pulmonary edema.

Situation 2 — Sarah Owens

In a patient like Mrs. Owens, daily body weights are the most accurate way to keep track of fluid status. Remember to weigh the patient daily, in the same kind of clothing, on the same scale, at the same time each day.

Situation 3

Aldosterone is normally inactivated by the liver. In some kinds of liver disease, aldosterone may not be properly degraded, resulting in sodium and water retention.

Situation 4 — Margaret Peters

Mrs. Peters' acidosis resulted from the use of Valium. The elderly are highly susceptible to respiratory depression with the use of sedatives. Such depression (hypoventilation) caused retention of carbon dioxide. The resulting rapid build-up of carbonic acid in the blood produced full-blown respiratory acidosis.

Situation 5 — Gerald James

Mr. James has probably had a massive shift of body fluid to the peritoneal cavity and abdominal tissues.

Common a few days after abdominal surgery, this resulted from peritoneal inflammation. His circulating blood volume is reduced and needs replacement with I.V. fluids. Such patients need careful monitoring of urine output, CVP, and vital signs to prevent volume overload as fluid shifts back into the circulation.

Situation 6 — Betty Lynn

Mrs. Lynn was hospitalized for full cardiac work-up (including EKG, echocardiogram for left ventricular function, chest X-ray, and blood work). None of the tests showed any deterioration from her previous cardiac work-up. Only her serum sodium had changed. It was high (148 mEq/L). Clearly her dyspnea was not due to further cardiac decompensation. Most likely, her emotional stress, due to menopause and her husband's problems, was stimulating increased release of ADH, causing increased water retention. She was also retaining sodium because of the estrogen. It was this combination of increased sodium and water retention that was causing her nocturnal dyspnea. Her estrogen was discontinued and furosemide was given to rid her of excess fluid. A tranquilizer was prescribed for her emotional stress. A social service consultant helped her husband find a job which eased his drinking problem. Mrs. Lynn's dyspnea disappeared.

Situation 7 — Mrs. Cooper

The nurse who discontinued the 3% NaCl realized that this solution is *hypertonic* and would have exceeded the patient's sodium requirements. Moreover, water restriction (usually to 25% to 50% of maintenance) is necessary when treating syndrome of inappropriate ADH (SIADH). If she had allowed this infusion to run, Mrs. Cooper would have gone into hypernatremia and convulsions, and may have died. Her nurse was correct in discontinuing the infusion and checking with the doctor for further orders. Infusions of saline solutions need careful monitoring of urinary output, vital signs, and serial electrolytes.

ANSWERS TO SKILLCHECK 3 (page 113)

Situation 1 — Sally Johnson

In metabolic acidosis, serum potassium levels are deceptively high. In an acidotic state, hydrogen ions enter the cells and are exchanged for potassium ions which leave the cell and enter the plasma. As acidosis is corrected, the potassium can rapidly shift back into the cell producing hypokalemia. So, watch for symptoms of hypokalemia as the blood sugar begins to return to normal. And keep intravenous potassium supplements handy since you will need to give potassium replacement.

Situation 2
These diuretics promote the excessive excretion of chloride ions and thus contribute to hypochloremic alkalosis.

Situation 3 — Mr. Puff
When a patient shifts so rapidly from respiratory acidosis to marked respiratory alkalosis, you can strongly suspect that he is being hyperventilated (in this case by the volume respirator). In respiratory alkalosis, serum calcium binds to the protein in blood with a resultant drop in serum calcium levels. Patients treated for acidosis sometimes overventilate and become alkalotic. If Mr. Puff's blood gases had been monitored more closely, appropriate changes in ventilator settings would have prevented alkalosis and hypocalcemia. The doctor was unaware at that time that Mr. Puff was on digitalis. A sudden increase in serum calcium levels in such a patient can precipitate digitalis toxicity as shown by Mr. Puff's atrial tachycardia with 2:1 block. Calcium must be given with extreme caution to patients on digitalis, with close monitoring of cardiac rhythms.

Situation 4 — Mr. Lloyd
Since the concentration of sodium is expressed as an amount per liter, the actual quantity of sodium is difficult to determine in this patient whose fluid status is so clearly deranged. Since he has not been eating or drinking normally for 5 days, he is probably just severely dehydrated. Once fluid volume is restored, his sodium level will probably return to normal.

Situation 5 — Ida Henry
If metastasis to the bone is indeed present, you should expect Mrs. Henry's serum calcium to be very high due to a shift of calcium from the bone to the serum. Initial treatment will probably consist of intravenous hydration with normal saline to prevent renal damage.

ANSWERS TO SKILLCHECK 4 (page 169)

Situation 1 — Mrs. Cramer
Mrs. Cramer's sudden and rapid change in mental status was probably caused by a shift in pH and rising PCO_2. Sedation in elderly patients with chronic obstructive pulmonary disease causes hypoventilation and an inability to blow off CO_2. Often, this causes hypercarbia, respiratory acidosis, and deranged sensorium. Call the doctor. Draw blood for blood gas evaluation and monitor the patient closely.

Situation 2 — Dwayne Marlin
The nurse who checked his chart found that Mr. Marlin had not been receiving his I.V. fluids at 6 ml/hour, but at about 20 ml/hour. He had also received a full 500 ml of fluid on his meal trays. In further assessing him, she noted distended neck veins, beginning bibasilar rales, sinus tachycardia, and an S_3 gallop. Oxygen by nasal cannula was started, and the doctor was notified that Mr. Marlin seemed to be going into congestive heart failure. It takes very little excess fluid to overload a patient such as Mr. Marlin. His I.V. should have been checked more carefully; his oral intake should have been watched to prevent exceeding his daily allowance. Obviously, too, his nurses should have checked the I.V., when he asked them to. If they had, they would have noticed fluid overload earlier. An I.V. monitor to control the infusion rate would also have helped. Still, the fundamental error in managing Mr. Marlin's care was inadequate monitoring by the nursing staff.

Situation 3 — Mr. Robinson
Chronic right-sided heart failure. This is probably due to his chronic left heart failure from his valvular heart disease. This causes increased resistance in the pulmonary system causing increasing pressure on the venous circulation.

Situation 4 — Robert Reed
Mr. Reed is in acidosis, probably of respiratory origin, since his PCO_2 is high. This condition is chronic, since his kidneys have had enough time to retain bicarbonate.

Situation 5 — Mrs. Lattimer
Report findings to doctor. Obviously, Mrs. Lattimer is retaining excess fluid despite diuretic treatment and has some degree of congestive heart failure. Reinforce the patient's salt intake and other dietary limitations. And check on visitors as a hidden source of salt. Patients get extra salt in candy bars and other gifts.

Situation 6 — Sarah Williams
As the kidneys begin to fail, they lose their ability to concentrate urine. In order to handle the usual load of urinary solutes, patients with renal insufficiency must drink and excrete more water than normal. Polyuria and polydipsia are, therefore, among the first signs of advancing renal failure.

ANSWERS TO SKILLCHECK 5 (page 195)

Situation 1 — Mr. Sealy
Try any of the following ways to dilate his veins:
• Lower his arm below his heart, i.e., down at his side.

- After applying the tourniquet, have the patient open and close his fist several times.
- With the tourniquet removed, apply warm compresses to his entire arm for at least 15 minutes.
- Gently tap or pat over the vein a few times. Remember, the resulting vein distention is short-lived, so be ready with your needle.

Situation 2
Your needle probably pierced the posterior wall of the vein causing a hematoma. This can happen because: You pierced the skin with the needle directly over top of the vein; the catheter and adapter were not securely held, causing accidental slipping; you selected a vein that has hard cover, rolls, or is thin and fragile (as in the elderly). The bedside table, particularly if on wheels, could also cause your hand and the needle to pitch forward unexpectedly during insertion and pierce the posterior wall of the vein.

Remove the needle and catheter and choose another site, keeping these things in mind. Also remember to remove the catheter and needle together to avoid needle damage and catheter emboli.

Situation 3 — Mrs. Teasdale
Answers c, d, and e are all correct.

Situation 4
When TPN solutions fall behind schedule, trying to catch up by increasing the drip rate adds a great concentration of glucose in too short a time. The drip rate should be increased only at the doctor's direction, and then, only by 10% of the original rate. Even this compensation should continue only until the time scheduled for the next bottle. Remember, increasing the drip rate also makes the patient vulnerable to fluid overload and consequently, congestive heart failure and pulmonary edema. If undetected, hyperglycemia causes osmotic diuresis and hyperosmolality, leading to dehydration, coma and death. Don't wait until signs of dehydration occur. Monitor fractional urine glucose *throughout* the day and serum glucose daily.

Situation 5
TPN is indicated in all of these situations. It is an important adjunct for any patient who is nutritionally depleted.

INDEX

SUGGESTED FURTHER READING

American College of Surgeons Committee on Pre & Postoperative Care. *Manual of Preoperative and Postoperative Care*. Philadelphia, W. B. Saunders, 1971.

Anthony, Catherine Parker. *Textbook of Anatomy and Physiology*. St. Louis, C. V. Mosby, 1975.

Ayres, Stephen, Stanley Giannelli, Hiltrud Mueller, and Meta E. Buehler. *Care of the Critically Ill*. New York, Appleton-Century-Crofts, 1975.

Brobeck, John R. *Best & Taylor's Physiological Basis of Medical Practice*. Baltimore, Williams & Wilkins, 1973.

Brunner, L. S., *et al. Lippincott Manual of Nursing Practice*. Philadelphia, J. B. Lippincott, 1978.

Brunner, L. S., *et al. Textbook of Medical Surgical Nursing*. St. Louis, C. V. Mosby, 1975.

Dillon, R. S. *Handbook of Endocrinology*. Philadelphia, Lea and Febiger, 1973.

Ezrin, E., J. O. Godden, and R. Volpe. *Systematic Endocrinology*. New York, Harper & Row, 1973.

Frohlich, Edward D. *Pathophysiology: Altered Regulatory Mechanisms in Disease*. Philadelphia, J. B. Lippincott, 1972.

Goldberger, Emanuel. *A Primer of Water, Electrolyte and Acid Base Syndromes*. Philadelphia, Lea & Febiger, 1975.

Goodman, L. S., and A. Gilman. *Pharmacological Basis of Therapeutics*. New York, Macmillan, 1975.

Guyton, Arthur C. *Textbook of Medical Physiology*. Philadelphia, W. B. Saunders, 1976.

Harrington, Joan, and Etta R. Brener. *Patient Care in Renal Failure*. Philadelphia, W. B. Saunders, 1973.

Jones, C. Archambeault, and I. Feller. *Procedures for Nursing the Burned Patient*. Ann Arbor, National Institute for Burn Medicine, 1975.

Kurdi, William. *Modern Intravenous Therapy Procedures*. California, Medical Education Consultants, 1976.

Leaf, A., and R. Cotran. *Renal Pathophysiology*. New York, Oxford University Press, 1976.

Lewis, LaVerne Wolff. *Fundamental Skills in Patient Care*. Philadelphia, J. B. Lippincott, 1976.

Luckmann, Joan, and Karen Sorensen. *Medical-Surgical Nursing: A Psychophysiologic Approach*. Philadelphia, W. B. Saunders, 1974.

Maude, D. L. *Kidney Physiology and Kidney Disease*. Philadelphia, J. B. Lippincott, 1977.

Maxwell, Morton H., and Charles R. Kleeman. *Clinical Disorders of Fluid & Electrolyte Metabolism*. New York, McGraw-Hill, 1972.

Metheney, Norma, and W. D. Snively. *Nurse's Handbook of Fluid Balance*. Philadelphia, J. B. Lippincott, 1974.

Netter, Frank. *The CIBA Collection of Medical Illustrations: Volume 6 – Kidneys, Ureters & Urinary Bladder*. New Jersey, CIBA Pharmaceuticals, 1974.

Papper, Solomon. *Clinical Nephrology*. Boston, Little, Brown, 1971.

Reed, Gretchen, and Vincent Sheppard. *Regulation of Fluid and Electrolyte Balance: A Programmed Instruction in Clinical Physiology*. Philadelphia, W. B. Saunders, 1977.

Samet, Phillip. *Cardiac Pacing*. New York, Grune & Stratton, 1973.

Schrier, Robert W. *Renal and Electrolyte Disorders*. Boston, Little, Brown, 1976.

Spencer, Roberta. *Patient Care in Endocrine Problems*. Philadelphia, W. B. Saunders, 1973.

Stroot, Violet, *et al. Fluid and Electrolytes*. Philadelphia, F. A. Davis, 1977.

Sweetwood, Hannelore. *The Patient in the Coronary Care Unit*. New York, Springer, 1976.

Thiele, Victoria. *Clinical Nutrition*. St. Louis, C. V. Mosby, 1976.

Waif, S. O. *Diabetes Mellitus*. Indianapolis, Lilly Research Labs, 1973.

Washington University Department of Medicine. *Manual of Medical Therapeutics*. Boston, Little, Brown, 1976.

Weldy, Norma Jean. *Body Fluids and Electrolytes: A Programmed Presentation*. St. Louis, C. V. Mosby, 1976.

Zimmerman, Clarence. *Techniques of Patient Care: A Manual of Bedside Procedures*. Boston, Little, Brown, 1976.